All rights Reserved. No part of this book may be reproduced or transmitted in any form by any means, graphic, electronic or mechanical including photocopying, recording, taping or by any information storage or retrieval system without written permission from publisher.

The purpose of this book is to inform, educate and entertain. Although every precaution has been taken in preparation of this book, there may be errors or omissions. Neither is any liability assumed for damages resulting, directly or indirectly, from the use of this information contained within this book.

Published by:

SureShot Books Publishing LLC
P.O. Box 924
Nyack, New York 10960

www.sureshotbooks.com

TABLE OF CONTENTS

PREFACE 1

ABOUT OBAMACARE 1

HIGHLIGHTS OF THE REGULATIONS UNDER
PRESIDENT OBAMA 2

OBAMACARE WANTS EVERYONE TO HAVE ACCESS TO
HEALTHCARE AND NOT ONLY THOSE WHO
CAN AFFORD IT 3

MYTHS ABOUT OBAMACARE 7

WHAT OBAMACARE PROVIDES 14

ACCESS TO THERAPIES 14

PERSONAL RESPONSIBILITY EDUCATION 15

    FAITH-BASED ORGANIZATIONS OR CONSORTIA. 15

        PERSONAL RESPONSIBILITY EDUCATION PROGRAMS 15

HEALTH CARE POWER OF ATTORNEY 16

    (a) INDEPENDENT LIVING EDUCATION. 16

TREATMENT OF CERTAIN COMPLEX DIAGNOSTIC
LABORATORY TESTS 16

MEDICAID 17

PREVENTION/WELLNESS 17

MEDICARE COVERAGE 18

WOMEN 18

PATIENT ACCESS TO OBSTETRICAL AND
GYNECOLOGICALCARE 18

ABORTION SERVICES 19

TABLE OF CONTENTS

COVERAGE FOR FREESTANDING BIRTH CENTER SERVICES *20*

FAMILY PLANNING SERVICES *21*

    RESTORATION OF FUNDING FOR ABSTINENCE EDUCATION *21*

ACTIVITIES REGARDING WOMEN'S HEALTH *22*

OFFICE OF WOMEN'S HEALTH *22*

PHSA IMMUNIZATIONS *23*

COVERAGE OF EMERGENCY SERVICES *23*

ACCESS TO PEDIATRIC CARE *24*

INFANTS, CHILDREN, ADOLESCENTS *25*

LONG TERM SERVICES AND SUPPPORT *25*

COMMUNITY FIRST CHOICE OPTION *25*

REMOVAL OF BARRIERS TO PROVIDING HOME AND COMMUNITY BASED SERVICES. *27*

PRESCRIPTION DRUG REBATES *27*

PROVIDING ADEQUATE PHARMACY REIMBURSEMENT *28*

STATE OPTION TO PROVIDE HEALTH HOMES FOR ENROLLEES WITH CHRONIC CONDITIONS *29*

DENTAL BENEFITS *29*

ADDITIONAL REQUIRED BENEFITS *30*

States may provide additional coverage. *30*

CONSUMER CHOICE *30*

LIFETIME OR ANNUAL LIMITS *31*

PROHIBITION ON RESCISSIONS *31*

TABLE OF CONTENTS

CONSUMER OPERATED PLANS *32*
ENSURING THE QUALITY OF CARE *34*
APPEALS PROCESS *34*
PREEXISTING CONDITION *35*
GUARANTEED AVAILABILITY OF COVERAGE *35*
GUARANTEED RENEWABILITY OF COVERAGE *36*
HEALTH STATUS *36*
PROGRAMS OF HEALTH PROMOTION OR DISEASE PREVENTION. *36*
    PROHIBITION ON EXCESSIVE WAITING PERIODS 37
CHOICE OF HEALTH CARE PROFESSIONAL *37*
ESSENTIAL BENEFITS *37*
CHANGES TO PRIVATE INSURANCE *38*
DEPENDENT COVERAGE *38*
INSURANCE MARKETS *38*
HEALTHCARE CHOICE COMPACTS *39*
ROLE OF STATES *40*
DUAL ELIGIBLES *41*
FRAUD AND ABUSE *41*
STATE FLEXIBILITY TO ESTABLISH ALTERNATIVE PROGRAMS *42*
PREMIUM TAX CREDITS AND COSTSHARING REDUCTIONS *44*
    REFUNDABLE CREDIT FOR COVERAGE UNDER A QUALIFIED HEALTH PLAN. 44
    ADDITIONAL BENEFITS 45

TABLE OF CONTENTS

SPECIAL RULE FOR PEDIATRIC DENTAL COVERAGE 45
RELIGIOUS EXEMPTIONS 45
HEALTH CARE SHARING MINISTRY 46
INDIVIDUALS WHO CANNOT AFFORD COVERAGE 46
FREEDOM NOT TO PARTICIPATE IN FEDERAL HEALTH INSURANCE PROGRAMS 46
NONDISCRIMINATION 47
PROTECTIONS FOR EMPLOYEES 47
SEC. 18C PROTECTIONS FOR EMPLOYEES 47
STATES MAY EXPAND ELIGIBILITY 48
MEDICAID MINIMUM BENEFITS 49
HOW TRUMP CARE HURTS AMERICANS 49
HOW WOULD REPEAL OF OBAMACARE AFFECT YOU 156
HEALTHCARE FOR PRISONERS 159
FAQ – CIVIL JUSTICE AND PRISON HEALTH CARE: ALL LOCKED UP AND BEHIND BARS 159
INDEX 165
REFERENCES 167

OBAMACARE-TRUMPCARE

PREFACE

I became interested in healthcare after Charles Ryan as Director of the Arizona Department Of Corrections denied me treatment for my serious medical needs, nearly killing me. They did this though Obamacare pays for this.[1]

I hope this guide will aid the reader in obtaining the maximum benefit from Obamacare.

ABOUT OBAMACARE

Fact Sheet[2]: Individual Shared Responsibility for Health Insurance Coverage and Minimum Essential Coverage Proposed Rules Under the Affordable Care Act, the Federal government, State governments, insurers, employers, and individuals are given shared responsibility to reform and improve the availability, quality, and affordability of health insurance coverage in the United States. Starting in 2014, the individual shared responsibility provision calls for each individual to have basic health insurance coverage (known as minimum essential coverage), qualify for an exemption, or make a shared responsibility payment when filing a federal income tax return. Individuals will not have to make a payment if coverage is unaffordable, if they spend less than three consecutive months without coverage, or if they qualify for an exemption for several other reasons, including hardship and religious beliefs.

Today, the Treasury Department and Internal Revenue Service (IRS), as well as the Centers for Medicare & Medicaid Services at the Department of Health and Human Services (HHS), issued two sets of proposed regulations. The regulations explain the shared responsibility provision and lay out the eligibility rules for receiving an exemption and the process by which individuals can receive certificates of exemption. Both agencies' proposed regulations include rules that will ease implementation and help to ensure that the payment applies only to the limited group of taxpayers who choose to spend a substantial period of time without coverage despite having ready access to affordable coverage.

According to the Congressional Budget Office, less than two percent of Americans will owe a shared responsibility payment.

HIGHLIGHTS OF THE REGULATIONS UNDER PRESIDENT OBAMA

A principle in implementing the individual shared responsibility provision is that the shared responsibility payment should not apply to any taxpayer for whom coverage is unaffordable, who has other good cause for going without coverage, or who goes without coverage for only a short time. The proposed regulations include several rules to implement this principle. For example:

Hardship Exemption Clarified to Protect Taxpayers, Address Key Concerns. The statute gives HHS authority to exempt individuals determined to "have suffered a hardship with respect to the capability to obtain coverage." In developing these proposed regulations, HHS considered several particular circumstances that provide good cause to go without coverage. To provide clarity for taxpayers facing these circumstances, the HHS proposed regulations enumerate several situations that will always be treated as constituting a hardship and therefore allow for an exemption. Hardship exemptions include:

o   Individuals whom an Exchange projects will have no offer of affordable coverage (even if, due to a change in circumstance during the year, it turns out that the coverage would have been affordable). This rule will protect individuals who turn down coverage because the Exchange projects itwill be unaffordable but whose actual income for the year turns out to be higher so they are not eligible for the affordability exemption;

o   Certain individuals who are not required to file an income tax return but who technically fall outside the statutory exemption for those with household income below the filing threshold; and

o   Individuals who would be eligible for Medicaid but for a state's choice not to expand Medicaid eligibility. This rule will protect individuals in states that, pursuant to the Supreme Court decision, choose not to expand Medicaid eligibility;

The HHS regulations also provide that the hardship exemption will be available on a case-by-case basis for individuals who face other unexpected personal or financial circumstances that prevent them from obtaining coverage.

Partial-Month Coverage Counts for the Month. The Treasury regulations provide that an individual is treated as having coverage for a month so long as he or she has coverage for any one day of that month. For example, an individual who starts a new job on March 27 and is enrolled in employer-sponsored coverage on that day is treated as having coverage for the month of March. Similarly, an individual who is eligible for an exemption for any one day of a month is treated as exempt for the entire month.

Payment Waived for First Part of Coverage Gap Spanning Multiple Years. The statute provides an exemption for gaps in coverage of less than three months. It generally specifies that such gaps be measured without regard to the calendar years in which the gap occurs. For example, a gap lasting from November through February lasts four months and therefore generally would not qualify for the exemption. However, recognizing that many individuals file their tax returns as early as January, before the length of an ongoing gap may be known, the Treasury regulations provide that if the part of a gap in the first tax year is less than three months, then no shared responsibility payment is due for the part of the gap that occurs during the first calendar year, regardless of the eventual length of the gap. For example, for a gap lasting from November through February, no payment would be due for November and December.

OBAMACARE WANTS EVERYONE TO HAVE ACCESS TO HEALTHCARE AND NOT ONLY THOSE WHO CAN AFFORD IT

SHAUN RICHMAN writes Obamacare[3] works by mandating that everyone get health insurance or pay a tax. Otherwise known as the Patient Protection and Affordable Care Act, it provides subsidies for middle-income families and small businesses. It pays for this by taxing some health care providers and high-income families. Medicare has also begun paying doctors for quality-of-care rather than on a fee-for-service basis. That will also lower health care costs and provide better health care for society as a whole.

In 2010, President Obama and Congress signed Obamacare into law. Why? They wanted to make sure all Americans were able to get health insurance. More important, they wanted to lower the cost of health care. That would reduce the growing cost of Medicare and Medicaid. Those two programs threaten to take over the entire federal budget.

The Act coordinates Federal health efforts around seven priority areas:
1. Tobacco-free living.
2. Preventing drug abuse and excessive alcohol use.
3. Healthy eating.
4. Active living.
5. Injury and violence-free living.
6. Reproductive and sexual health.
7. Mental and emotional health.

The Act funds scholarships and loans to increase the number of primary care physicians, nurses, physician assistants, mental health providers, and dentists. Its goal is to double the number of patients treated in five years.

The Act requires doctors to report on any financial interest they have with imaging companies, etc., and provide a list of alternative service providers to patients. It requires medical device makers, drug companies, etc., to reveal financial arrangements they have with doctors. Enterprises that manage the prescription drug portion of Medicare or the state exchanges are required to report any financial concessions they receive from pharmaceutical companies.

The Act provides training and requires background checks for nursing home staff to reduce elder abuse.

It also cracks down on fraud by identifying high-risk providers and preventing them from setting up in another state. It gives states the ability to test legal reforms to enhance patient safety, encourage efficient resolution of disputes, and improve access to liability insurance.

The Act gives drug discounts to hospitals that serve low-income patients. It also requires competitive pricing for vaccines and hormone therapies.

The CLASS Act allowed Americans who are or become physically challenged to receive a $50 daily payment to put toward assisted living. They must pay premiums for five years, and work for three of those years. The amount went toward home health care, adult day care, and other services to allow them to stay in their homes. It also went toward assisted living facilities, nursing homes, and group homes. It was self-funded. It would have reduced the deficit by $70.2 billion over ten years.

OBAMACARE-TRUMPCARE

It would have allowed people to keep working and stay out of nursing homes and the hospital. It entered into force on January 1, 2011, but by October 1 it was determined to be unworkable. It could not compete with private sector plans that offered better benefits.

Going to the doctor or the hospital has become very expensive. In fact, health care costs are the No. 1 cause of bankruptcy in this country.

Just one visit to the emergency room costs $1,265 on average. A broken foot costs around $16,000, while cancer treatment can cost $30,000. For more, see Health care Blue Book.

People with health insurance don't have to worry about these costs since their insurance pays most of them. The insured only pay a small fee per visit, called a copayment. Most people get health insurance as a benefit from their employer. The company usually pays part of the monthly cost, known as a premium.

Some of them are poor enough to qualify for Medicaid, paid for by state and federal governments. Those who are older than 65 receive Medicare. They pay premiums that the federal government subsidizes.

People who make too much money for Medicaid and are too young for Medicare, but are self-employed or don't get insurance from their jobs have to pay for their insurance, and it's very expensive. Before Obamacare, many just did without it and took their chances. Some had a chronic illness, called a "pre-existing condition," and the insurance companies wouldn't even offer them coverage.

There were anywhere from 32 million to 50 million people who didn't have health insurance.

If something happened and they had to go to the hospital, they often just didn't pay the bill. The hospital charged it to an emergency Medicaid plan. That raised the cost of health care for everyone.

Its aim is simple - to extend health insurance coverage to some of the estimated 15% of the US population who lack it. Those people receive no coverage from their employers and are not covered by US health programmes for the poor and elderly.

To achieve this, the law requires all Americans to have health insurance, but offers subsidies to make coverage more affordable and aims to reduce the cost of insurance by bringing younger, healthier people into the medical coverage system.

It also requires businesses with more than 50 full-time employees to offer health insurance.

The law creates state-run marketplaces - with websites akin to online travel and shopping sites - where individuals can compare prices as they shop for coverage. Some states have chosen not to participate in the ACA, and their residents can shop on a marketplace run by the federal government.

In addition, the law bans insurance companies from denying health coverage to people with pre-existing health conditions, allows young people to remain on their parents' plans until age 26, and expands eligibility for the government-run Medicaid health programme for the poor.

The law aims eventually to slow the growth of US healthcare spending, which is the highest in the world.

Obamacare should lower premiums over time by reducing health care and insurance costs. It requires everyone to have insurance for nine months out of the year. It allows parents to add their children up to age 26. As a result, more young, healthy people pay premiums but don't use the system, adding to health insurance companies' profits. The competitive insurance marketplace provides incentives for businesses to pass these savings on to customers through lower premiums. This would change if Trump Replaces Obamacare. People With Health Insurance - Here's six ways Obamacare improves your family's health insurance.

1. Parents can add their adult children (up to age 26) to their plans.
2. If anyone gets sick, the insurance company can't drop them from the plan or limit how much insurance your family uses.
3. If anyone is chronically ill, a new insurance company can't deny coverage.
4. Wellness and pregnancy exams are now free. That includes copayments.
5. Insurance companies can't raise premium payments without approval from state governments.
6. Some families received a check from the insurance company. That's because Obamacare says that companies must spend at least 80 percent of premiums on providing actual medical services. If they spent it on advertising or executive salaries, they have to pay the excess back to policy-holders.

Similarly, Obamacare subsidizes prescriptions for those on Medicare. This allows seniors to continue taking medications and prevent emergency room visits, further lowering the cost of insurance.

Health insurance plans are sold on the health insurance exchanges from November through January each year.

You can always use the exchanges to compare health plans and find out if you qualify for tax credits or subsidies. You can also use them to see if you are eligible for expanded Medicaid, which you can get any time of the year.

Each exchange uses a four-step process:

1. Create an account. It asks you several personal questions to verify your identity.
2. Provide Social Security and income information to see if you qualify for tax credits.
3. Review plans in the four categories (Bronze, Silver, Gold and Platinum). Each category has different monthly premiums, deductibles and co pays. Here's how health insurance works.
4. Enroll in the plan.

The federal government manages the exchanges in about half the states. These exchanges were difficult to get into at first but work fine now. The remaining states have either created their own exchanges or partnered with the federal government.

The exchanges allow you to compare physicians, hospitals, nursing homes, home health agencies and dialysis services.

MYTHS ABOUT OBAMACARE

The ACA affects everyone differently.

Myth 1: Health insurance costs are rising thanks to Obamacare.

Truth: Health insurance premiums have been rising, but not because of the ACA.

Premiums for company-sponsored family plans, for example, increased 4.8 percent annually between 2005 – 2010. Since the ACA was enacted, they've gone up at a slower rate of 3.8 percent a year.

Premiums for privately-bought plans rose 15 – 20 percent a year between 2005 - 2010. In 2013, the health insurance exchanges opened, and 39 percent experienced an increase. But 46 percent of enrollees saw lower premiums.

Many people across the board experienced higher rates because their plans now had to add the 10 essential health benefits. But health insurance costs were rising even without Obamacare.

Myth 2: Under Obamacare, you are forced to pay higher premiums for services you don't need, such as pregnancy, childbirth, and maternity care.

Truth: In any health insurance plan, someone is paying for services they know they'll never need. A marathoner will never need diabetes care; women will never need prostate testing, etc. Obamacare requires childbirth coverage to lower overall health care costs. That's because Medicaid pays for 50 percent of all childbirths.

It costs the taxpayer less to make sure those women receive prenatal care. That is cheaper than the emergency room treatment that results from botched home deliveries.

Myth 3: Obamacare is socialized medicine, like in Canada or the United Kingdom.

Truth: Not really. In the UK, doctors are employees of the federal government. In Canada, the government pays most medical bills. That's similar to America's Medicare and Medicaid. The ACA does expand Medicaid to middle-income families, but most of the expansion is in the private insurance market.

Why do more than half (57 percent) of Americans think the ACA is socialized medicine? President Obama's initial proposal included government-funded health coverage for Congress. Congress rejected his proposal. Ironically, Obamacare now forces Congress onto the private exchange, just like everyone else. So, in that particular case, the ACA is reducing socialized medicine.

Myth 4: President Obama promised that "If you like your plan, you can keep your plan, period." He meant that the ACA itself did not cancel anyone's plans. It also allowed plans to be "grandfathered in" if they existed before the ACA was passed.

That's as long as certain minimal requirements were met.

Truth: One million people lost their plans because their insurance companies dropped them. Some companies that didn't comply with the ACA's requirements chose to drop plans rather than change them. Even some "grandfathered in" policies were dropped. In 2014, Kaiser Permanente canceled "grandfathered in" policies for 3,414 customers in

Maryland and Virginia. Humana did the same for 6,544 plans in Kentucky. They decided it didn't make business sense to maintain a broad variety of plans at different costs.

Many employees lost their plans because their companies decided to pay the penalty. They knew their workers could find cheaper plans on the exchanges

Myth 5: Obamacare intrudes into the doctor-patient relationship by allowing government bureaucrats to decide your treatment, not your doctor.

Truth: Your relationship with your doctor hasn't changed. Bureaucrats have always been involved. Your doctor decides on the treatment. Then, an insurance company staff person decides whether it will be covered. That person also decides how much will be covered and how much the doctor will be paid for it. For Medicare and Medicare, the government is involved in this decision by acting as the insurance company. The ACA didn't change any of this.

Myth 6: Obamacare cuts benefits for those on Medicare.

Truth: Benefits aren't cut, although 44 percent of people believe they are. That's because the ACA cuts funding for Medicare by $716 billion over ten years. The cuts affect providers in these three areas:

Hospitals receive $260 billion less because the ACA changes the way they are paid. Before, they were payed "fee-for-service" for every test and procedure. Now they're switching to value-based care. This pays based on successful outcomes. You should receive better care at a lower cost.

Medicare Advantage insurance providers receive $156 billion less. This is because the ACA restricts cost increases to one percent above the rate of economic growth. Plans had risen 5.9 percent a year over the last five years, costing enrollees 17 percent more than regular plans. Home health care, skilled nursing services and hospice receive the rest of the cuts.

The ACA increased Medicare benefits. Medicare now includes free preventive care, like physicals and mammograms. In 2020, beneficiaries will receive 100 percent funding for the Part D "doughnut hole" prescription drug costs.

Myth 7: All your personal and medical information will be combined into a giant database. That will allow the government to keep better track of you.

Truth: The health insurance exchanges ask for a lot of personal data. You need to enter things like your Social Security number, your income and whether you smoke. The IRS uses this data to check against its records to make sure you qualify for the subsidy. The smoking question is because insurance companies can charge more for smokers. The government has most of this info already.

The ACA requires health care providers to computerize their records. This could one day be connected to the info on the exchanges. Could a despot use this database to control your life? Probably, but there is already so much data about you that your privacy is already compromised.

Myth 8: My tax dollars go toward providing immigrants who are in the country illegally with free health insurance.

Truth: Almost half (47 percent) agree with this statement. In fact, immigrants in the country illegally are prohibited from getting Obamacare. They can get preventive care at community health centers. That is supposed to lower health care costs. As before the ACA, emergency rooms must treat everyone. When more people in the country illegally use community health centers, there are fewer expensive emergency room bills.

Myth 9: Obamacare's childbirth coverage benefits makes people come to the United States so their children will be American citizens. These "anchor babies" make it easier for the parents to become citizens themselves.

Truth: Hospitals must treat anyone who shows up in the emergency room. Medicaid refunds around $2 billion a year to hospitals that treat at least 100,000 people here without legal permission. California alone receives $1 billion. But this existed before the ACA. Does it create an incentive for people without documentation to give birth in the United States? Maybe, but it's more likely that the primary motivation is jobs. That's clear because there were fewer people here illegally during the recession when jobs were scarce.

Myth 10: Businesses aren't hiring because of Obamacare.

Truth: The requirement to provide insurance affects only a few companies. More than 95 percent of companies with more than 50 employees already offered insurance. Of those that didn't, only 10 percent said they are reducing their workforce, cutting their hours or hiring more part-time, temporary or contract workers to avoid the requirement. Businesses with fewer than 50 employees are exempt. Those small companies create 65 percent of all new jobs

Myth 11: The Affordable Care Act is much better than Obamacare.

Truth: They are two names for the same thing. Many people think they are different. Forty-five percent of Americans polled in a 2012 Gallup poll approved of the ACA, while only 38 percent approved of Obamacare.

Myth 12: Most Americans think that Obamacare should be repealed.

Truth: More than half (54 percent) of Americans are opposed to Obamacare. But only 35 percent think it should be abolished. Sixteen percent believe it's too conservative. Twelve percent think it's already been repealed, and 7 percent think the Supreme Court ruled against it.

Myth 13: Obamacare established "death panels" that allow the government to make decisions about end-of-life care for people on Medicare.

Truth: The ACA initially proposed that Medicare provides 100 percent free coverage for doctor appointments with recipients who wanted to discuss do-not-resuscitate orders, end-of-life directives and living wills. Thanks to the controversy, the provision was dropped. Forty percent of people believe it exists.

Myth 14: The ACA creates "Taxmageddon," a massive tax increase of $800 billion over the next 10 years.

Truth: Obamacare tax increases will take in $76.8 billion a year when they are all up and running. That's the highest amount in history. It does slow economic growth at a dangerous time in the business cycle. The next largest increase was the 1993 deficit reduction bill. It raised $65.9 billion a year. The 1982 tax hike is third. But this doesn't take into account inflation, population growth, income growth and economic growth.

If you take inflation into account, then the 1982 tax increase was the largest, bringing in $85.3 billion. If you compare the tax increase as a percent of the total economy, then the 1942 tax increase to fund World War II was the largest. It was 5.04 percent of total economic output. That's over ten times larger than the 0.43 percent for the ACA.

If you had your plan before March 23, 2010, Obamacare allows you to keep it even if it doesn't comply. That means your plan might not have the ten 10 essential benefits. Many of those plans were "grandfathered in" and are exempt from Obamacare.

But your plan may have been canceled by the insurance company or by your employer. Obamacare's real promise is that if you lose your health care plan, you can get a new one. No insurer can turn you away because of health or age, and you'll be able to get financial help if you need it. Here's where to start.

I Have a Company Plan - You can keep it. You still may want to comparison shop on the exchanges. Some companies might find it more - effective to pay the penalty, knowing their workers can get coverage on the exchanges. Others found out their plans didn't provide the 10 essential benefits. In fact, 3 million to 5 million employees might lose their existing plans for this reason.

I Have Private Insurance - If it's an individual plan you bought yourself, you can keep it. But compare it to the plans on the exchanges to see if you can get better coverage at a lower price. You might also qualify to get subsidies if you buy a plan on the exchange.

I Have a Vision Care or Dental Discount Plan, other Discount Plan or Workers' Comp - You need to buy insurance on the exchange. These plans are not the same as health insurance. Find out How to Get Obamacare.

I Have Catastrophic Insurance - You can keep it. You may want to shop for a full-coverage plan on the exchange. But if you give up your catastrophic insurance you won't be able to go back. All insurance purchased after January 1, 2014, must have minimum benefits. Catastrophic insurance will only be available in certain circumstances.

I Have Medicare - You can stay on Medicare. If you have Medicare Part D, Obamacare helps pay for your prescription drugs if you fall into the "doughnut hole." By 2020, the ACA will eliminate the doughnut hole.

I Have Medicaid - You can stay on Medicaid.

I Have Other Insurance - You can keep most other plans, including retiree plans, CHIP, TRICARE and other veterans' health care programs, as well as Peace Corps Volunteer plans. See qualifying health plans here.
I Don't Have Insurance

If you didn't have insurance for at least nine months this year, you would have to pay extra on your income tax. To find out how much, see Obamacare Taxes.

OBAMACARE-TRUMPCARE

I Can't Afford Insurance - If your income is 138 percent or less of the federal poverty level, you qualify for Medicaid if your state agreed to expand coverage. If your state didn't agree, you wouldn't have to pay the tax. Find out more about Medicaid. See if you qualify for Medicaid.

If your income is under 400 percent of the poverty level, you can get a tax credit and possibly reduced copayments and deductibles.

I'm Unemployed - If you have COBRA, you can keep it. But you may want to shop the health care exchanges to see if you can get a better deal. Find out more. If you have no insurance, you may qualify for Medicaid or subsidies, depending on your family's income.

I Don't Need Insurance - If you are healthy, you may find it less expensive to pay the tax, depending on your income. Find low-cost community health centers in your area.

I Don't Want Insurance - You must pay the tax, as well as any health care costs. If you remain healthy, that's great. But keep in mind that the average emergency room visit is $1,265, while a broken leg can cost twice as much. Cancer treatment can cost $30,000 ($7,000 for chemotherapy alone). Like homeowners or car insurance, health insurance is designed to protect your life savings.

I Need Insurance Now - The exchanges can help you shop for medical care providers and private insurance now. You won't be eligible for subsidies or tax credits until next year. Compare plans now.

I'm a Small Business Owner

25 employees or less - You may already be eligible for a tax credit of 35 percent of the insurance you provide.

50 employees or less - You can use the exchange to find the best insurance.

50 or more employees - You must provide affordable health insurance that provides minimum value or pay a tax of $2,000 per employee (for all but the first 30 employees). If a worker finds a lower-cost plan on the exchange, you may be taxed.

If you offer health insurance as a benefit to early retirees ages 55 to 64, you can get federal financial assistance.

I'm a Member or Staff of Congress

You must get health insurance through the exchanges, instead of the government-provided health insurance you get now. You will continue to receive $4,900 ($10,000 for families) to help pay for your coverage

It's estimated that 22 million would lose medical insurance if Obamacare were repealed. Provisions of the law make care accessible to those who had previously been shut out. The uninsured rate has dropped by 5% since the programme began.

Some of the more popular provisions include:

- Children can stay on their parent's health care plan until age 26
- No one can be denied insurance for a pre-existing medical condition
- Companies can no longer charge women more than men

Require the Office of Personnel Management to contract with insurers to offer at least two multi-state plans in each Exchange. At least one plan must be offered by a non-profit entity and at least one plan must not provide coverage for abortions beyond those permitted by federal law. Each multi-state plan must be licensed in each state and must meet the qualifications of a qualified health plan. If a state has lower age rating requirements than 3:1, the state may require multi-state plans to meet the more protective age rating rules. These multi-state plans will be offered separately from the Federal Employees Health Benefit Program and will have a separate risk pool.

WHAT OBAMACARE PROVIDES

ACCESS TO THERAPIES

Notwithstanding any other provision of this Act, the Secretary[4] of Health and Human Services shall not promulgate any regulation that—

(1) creates any unreasonable barriers to the ability of individuals to obtain appropriate medical care;

(2) impedes timely access to health care services;

(3) interferes with communications regarding a full range of treatment options between the patient and the provider;

(4) restricts the ability of health care providers to provide full disclosure of all relevant information to patients making health care decisions;

(5) violates the principles of informed consent and the ethical standards of health care professionals; or

(6) limits the availability of health care treatment for the full duration of a patient's medical needs.

WHAT THIS MEANS

Therapy assistance is to be provided.

PERSONAL RESPONSIBILITY EDUCATION

FAITH-BASED ORGANIZATIONS OR CONSORTIA.

The Secretary may solicit and award grants under this⁵paragraph to faith-based organizations or consortia.

PERSONAL RESPONSIBILITY EDUCATION PROGRAMS. Personal responsibility education program means a program that is designed to educate adolescents on (i) both abstinence and contraception for the prevention of pregnancy and sexually transmitted infections, including HIV/AIDS, consistent with the requirements. IT IS NECESSARY (i) The program replicates evidence-based effective programs or substantially incorporates elements of effective programs that have been proven on the basis of rigorous scientific research to change behavior, which means delaying sexual activity, increasing condom or contraceptive use for sexually active youth, or reducing pregnancy among youth. (ii) The program is medically-accurate and complete. (iii) The program includes activities to educate youth who are sexually active regarding responsible sexual behavior with respect to both abstinence and the use of contraception. (iv) The program places substantial emphasis on both abstinence and contraception for the prevention of pregnancy among youth and sexually transmitted infections. (v) The program provides age-appropriate information and activities. (vi) The information and activities carried out under the program are provided in the cultural context that is most appropriate for individuals in the particular population group to which they are directed.

(C) **ADULTHOOD PREPARATION SUBJECTS.**—The adulthood preparation subjects are the following: (i) Healthy relationships, including marriage and family interactions. (ii) Adolescent development, such as the development of healthy attitudes and values about adolescent growth and development, body image, racial and ethnic diversity, and other related subjects. (iii) Financial literacy. (iv) Parent-child communication. (v) Educational and career success, such as developing skills for employment preparation, job seeking, independent living, financial self-sufficiency, and workplace productivity. (vi) Healthy life skills, such as goal-setting, decision making, negotiation, communication and interpersonal skills, and stress management.

HEALTH CARE POWER OF ATTORNEY

The importance of designating another individual[6] to make health care treatment decisions on behalf of the child if

the child becomes unable to participate in such decisions and the child does not have, or does not want, a relative who would otherwise be authorized under State law to make such decisions, and provides the child with the option to execute a health care power of attorney, health care proxy, or other similar document recognized under State law," after "employment services,".

> (a) **INDEPENDENT LIVING EDUCATION.** (K) A certification by the chief executive officer of the State that the State will ensure that an adolescent participating in the program under this section are provided with education about the importance of designating another individual to make health care treatment decisions on behalf of the adolescent if the adolescent becomes unable to participate in such decisions and the adolescent does not have, or does not want, a relative who would otherwise be authorized under State law to make such decisions, whether a health care power of attorney, health care proxy, or other similar document is recognized under State law, and how to execute such a document if the adolescent wants to do so.

TREATMENT OF CERTAIN COMPLEX DIAGNOSTIC LABORATORY TESTS

DEMONSTRATION PROJECT (1) IN GENERAL separate payments are made under such part for complex diagnostic laboratory tests [7]provided to individuals for tests (A) that is an analysis of gene protein expression, topographic genotyping, or a cancer chemotherapy sensitivity assay; (B) that is determined by the Secretary to be a laboratory test for which there is not an alternative test having equivalent performance characteristics; (C) which is billed using a Health Care Procedure Coding System (HCPCS) code other than a not otherwise classified code under such Coding System; (D) which is approved or cleared by the Food and Drug Administration or is covered under title XVIII of the Social Security Act; and (E) is described in section 1861(s)(3) of the Social Security Act (42 U.S.C. 1395x(s)(3)).

WHAT THIS MEANS

Expensive and complex tests are covered.

MEDICAID

Create a new Medicaid state plan option to permit Medicaid enrollees with at least two chronic conditions, one condition and risk of developing another, or at least one serious and persistent mental health condition to designate a provider as a home health. Provide states taking up the option with 90% FMAP for two years for home health-related services, including care management, care coordination, and health promotion. Expand the role of the Medicaid and CHIP Payment and Access Commission to include assessments of adult services (including those dually eligible for Medicare and Medicaid.

WHAT THIS MEANS

Medicaid enrollees with at least two chronic conditions, one condition and risk of developing another, or at least one serious and persistent mental health may designate a provider as a home health if states allow.

PREVENTION/WELLNESS

Establish the National Prevention, Health Promotion and Public Health Council to coordinate federal prevention, wellness, and public health activities. Develop a national strategy to improve the nation's health.

WHAT THIS MEANS

Provide incentives to Medicare and Medicaid beneficiaries to complete behavior modification programs. Require qualified health plans to provide at a minimum coverage without cost-sharing for preventive services rated A or B by the U.S. Preventive Services Task Force, recommended immunizations, preventive care for infants, children, and adolescents, and additional preventive care and screenings for women.

Those on Medicaid and Medicare receive education on immunizations, preventive care for infants, children, and adolescents, and additional preventive care and screenings for women.

MEDICARE COVERAGE

Expand Medicare coverage to individuals who have been exposed to environmental health hazards from living in an area subject to an emergency declaration made as of June 17, 2009 and have developed certain health conditions as a result.

WHAT THIS MEANS

Those exposed to environmental health hazards from living in an area subject to an emergency declaration made as of June 17, 2009 and have developed certain health conditions as a result are covered.

WOMEN

With respect to women, such additional preventive care and screenings not described in paragraph (1) as provided for in comprehensive guidelines supported by the Health Resources and Services Administration for purposes of this paragraph. 5) Breast cancer screening, mammography, and prevention shall be considered the most current.

WHAT THIS MEANS

For women preventive care and Breast cancer screening, mammography, and prevention shall be covered.

PATIENT ACCESS TO OBSTETRICAL AND GYNECOLOGICALCARE

(d) (1) (A) DIRECT ACCESS.—A group health plan, or health insurance issuer offering group or individual health insurance coverage, described in paragraph (2) may not require authorization or referral by the plan, issuer, or any person (including a primary care provider described in paragraph (2)(B)) in the case of a female participant, beneficiary, or enrollee who seeks coverage for obstetrical or gynecological care provided by a participating health care professional who specializes in obstetrics or gynecology. Such professional shall agree to otherwise adhere to such plan's or issuer's policies and procedures, including procedures regarding referrals and obtaining prior authorization and providing services pursuant to a treatment plan (if any) approved by the plan or issuer.

WHAT THIS MEANS

Obstetrical or gynecological care is to be provided.

ABORTION SERVICES

(b) SPECIAL RULES RELATING TO COVERAGE OF
(1) VOLUNTARY CHOICE OF COVERAGE OF ABORTION SERVICES (A) IN GENERAL. (i) nothing in this title (or any amendment made by this title), shall be construed to require a qualified health plan to provide coverage of services described in subparagraph (B)(i) or (B)(ii) as part of its essential health benefits for any plan year; and (ii) subject to subsection (a), the issuer of a qualified health plan shall determine whether or not the plan provides coverage of services described in subparagraph (B)(i) or (B)(ii) as part of such benefits for the plan year.
(B) (i) ABORTIONS FOR WHICH PUBLIC FUNDING IS PROHIBITED. The services described in this clause are abortions for which the expenditure of Federal funds appropriated for the Department of Health and Human Services is not permitted, based on the law as in effect as of the date that is 6 months before the beginning of the plan year involved.
(ii) ABORTIONS FOR WHICH PUBLIC FUNDING IS ALLOWED. The services described in this clause are abortions for which the expenditure of Federal funds appropriated for the Department of Health and Human Services is permitted, based on the law as in effect as of the date that is 6 months before the beginning of the plan year involved.
Permit states to prohibit plans participating in the Exchange from providing coverage for abortions.
Require plans that choose to offer coverage for abortions beyond those for which federal funds are permitted (to save the life of the woman and in cases of rape or incest) in states that allow such coverage to create allocation accounts for segregating premium payments for coverage of

abortion services from premium payments for coverage for all other services to ensure that no federal premium or cost-sharing subsidies are used to pay for the abortion coverage. Plans must also estimate the actuarial value of covering abortions by taking into account the cost of the abortion benefit (valued at no less than $1 per enrollee per month) and cannot take into account any savings that might be reaped as a result of the abortions. Prohibit plans participating in the Exchanges from discriminating against any provider because of unwillingness to provide, pay for, provide coverage of, or refer for abortions.

WHAT THIS MEANS

ABORTIONS are to be covered but federal funds must not be used.

Plans that choose coverage for abortions beyond those for which federal funds are permitted (to save the life of the woman and in cases of rape or incest) in states that allow such coverage to create allocation accounts for segregating premium payments for coverage of abortion services

COVERAGE FOR FREESTANDING BIRTH CENTER SERVICES

(a) (28) freestanding birth center services[8] and other ambulatory services that are offered by a freestanding birth center and that are otherwise included in the plan; and"; and

(3)(A) The term 'freestanding birth center services' means services furnished to an individual at a freestanding birth center (as defined in subparagraph (B)) at such center.

(B) The term 'freestanding birth center' means a health facility —

(i) that is not a hospital;

(ii) where childbirth is planned to occur away from the pregnant woman's residence;

(iii) that is licensed or otherwise approved by the State to provide prenatal labor and delivery or postpartum care and

other ambulatory services that are included in the plan; and

(iv) that complies with such other requirements relating to the health and safety of individuals furnished services by

the facility as the State shall establish.

(C) A State shall provide separate payments to providers administering prenatal labor and delivery or postpartum care in a freestanding birth center (as defined in subparagraph (B)), such as nurse midwives and other providers of services such as birth attendants recognized under State law, as determined appropriate by the Secretary. For purposes of the preceding sentence, the term 'birth attendant' means an individual who is recognized or registered by the State involved to provide health care at childbirth and who provides such care within the scope of practice under which the individual is legally authorized to perform such care under State law (or the State regulatory mechanism provided by State law), regardless of whether the individual is under the supervision of, or associated with, a physician or other health care provider. Nothing in this subparagraph shall be construed as changing State law requirements applicable to a birth attendant.

WHAT THIS MEANS

Freestanding birth center services and other ambulatory services that are offered by a freestanding birth center is covered.

FAMILY PLANNING SERVICES

(a) STATE OPTION. — State plan approved under section 1902 may provide for making medical⁹assistance available to an individual described in section 1902(ii) (relating to individuals who meet certain income eligibility standard)

during a presumptive eligibility period. In the case of an individual described in section 1902(ii), such medical assistance shall be limited to family planning services and supplies described in 1905(a)(4)(C) and, at the State's option, medical diagnosis and treatment services that are provided in conjunction with a family planning service in a family planning setting.

(7) COVERAGE OF FAMILY PLANNING SERVICES AND SUPPLIES. A State may not provide for medical assistance through enrollment of an individual with benchmark coverage or benchmark-equivalent coverage under this section unless such coverage includes for any individual described in section 1905(a)(4)(C), medical assistance for family planning services and supplies in accordance with such section.

WHAT THIS MEANS

Family planning services is covered if states wish to provide the coverage.

RESTORATION OF FUNDING FOR ABSTINENCE EDUCATION [10]

Obamacare provides funds for patients to be taught abstinence.

ACTIVITIES REGARDING WOMEN'S HEALTH

(a) ESTABLISHMENT. — There is established within the Office of the Director, an Office of Women's Health and Gender-Based Research (referred to in this section as the 'Office'). The Office shall be headed by a director who shall be appointed by the Director of Healthcare and Research Quality.

(b) PURPOSE. — The official designated under subsection (a) shall —

(1) report to the Director on the current Agency level of activity regarding women's health, across, where appropriate, age, biological, and sociocultural contexts, in all aspects of Agency work, including the development of evidence reports and clinical practice protocols and the conduct of research into patient outcomes, delivery of health care services, quality of care, and access to health care;

(2) establish short-range and long-range goals and objectives within the Agency for research important to women's[11]

health and, as relevant and appropriate, coordinate with other appropriate offices on activities within the Agency that relate to health services and medical effectiveness research, for issues of particular concern to women;

(3) identify projects in women's health that should be conducted or supported by the Agency;

(4) consult with health professionals, nongovernmental organizations, consumer organizations, women's health professionals, and other individuals and groups, as appropriate, on Agency policy with regard to women; and

(5) serve as a member of the Department of Health and Human Services Coordinating Committee on Women's Health (established under section 229(b)(4)).

OFFICE OF **WOMEN'S** HEALTH [12]

Consult with health professionals, nongovernmental organizations, consumer organizations, women's health professionals, and other individuals and groups, as appropriate, on Administration policy with regard to women;

(1) report to the Commissioner of Food and Drugs on current Food and Drug Administration (referred to in this section as the

'Administration') levels of activity regarding women's participation in clinical trials and the analysis of data by sex in the testing of drugs, medical devices, and biological products across, where appropriate, age, biological, and sociocultural contexts;

(3) provide information to women and health care providers on those areas in which differences between men and women exist;

(4) consult with pharmaceutical, biologics, and device manufacturers, health professionals with expertise in women's issues, consumer organizations, and women's health professionals on Administration policy with regard to women;

PHSA IMMUNIZATIONS

Immunizations that have in effect a recommendation from the Advisory Committee on Immunization Practices of the Centers for Disease Control and Prevention with respect to the individual involved;[13]

WHAT THIS MEANS

Immunizations are covered.

COVERAGE OF EMERGENCY SERVICES

If a group health plan, or a health insurance issuer offering group or individual health insurance issuer, provides or covers any benefits with respect to services in an emergency department of a hospital, the plan or issuer shall cover emergency services.

(A) Without the need for any prior authorization determination;

(B) Whether the health care provider furnishing such services is a participating provider with respect to such services;

(C) In a manner so that, if such services are provided to a participant, beneficiary, or enrollee—

(i) By a nonparticipating health care provider with or without prior authorization; or

(ii)(I) Such services will be provided without imposing any requirement under the plan for prior authorization of services or any limitation on coverage where the provider of services does not have a contractual relationship with the plan for the providing of services that is more restrictive than the requirements or limitations that apply to emergency department services received from providers who do have such a contractual relationship with the plan; and

(II) If such services are provided out-of-network, the cost-sharing requirement (expressed as a copayment amount or coinsurance rate) is the same requirement that would apply if such services were provided in-network;

(2) (A) **EMERGENCY MEDICAL CONDITION.**—The term 'emergency medical condition' means a medical condition manifesting itself by acute symptoms of sufficient severity (including severe pain) such that a prudent layperson, who possesses an average knowledge of health and medicine, could reasonably expect the absence of immediate medical attention.

(B) EMERGENCY SERVICES.—The term 'emergency services' means, with respect to an emergency medical condition—

(i) a medical screening examination (as required under section 1867 of the Social Security Act) that is within the capability of the emergency department of a hospital, including ancillary services routinely available to the emergency department to evaluate such emergency medical condition, and

(ii) within the capabilities of the staff and facilities available at the hospital, such further medical examination and treatment as are required under section 1867 of such Act to stabilize the patient.

WHAT THIS MEANS

Emergency care is covered.

ACCESS TO PEDIATRIC CARE

(c)(1) In the case of a person who has a child who is a participant, beneficiary, or enrollee under a group health plan, or health insurance coverage offered by a health insurance issuer in the group or individual market, if the plan or issuer requires or provides for the designation of a participating primary care provider for the child, the plan or issuer shall permit such person to designate a physician (allopathic or osteopathic) who specializes in pediatrics as the child's primary care provider if such provider participates in the network of the plan or issuer.

WHAT THIS MEANS

Plans must provide care for children.

INFANTS, CHILDREN, ADOLESCENTS

With respect to infants, children, and adolescents, evidence-informed preventive care and screenings provided for in the comprehensive guidelines supported by the Health Resources and Services Administration.

WHAT THIS MEANS

Preventive care and screenings to infants, children, and adolescents are covered.

LONG TERM SERVICES AND SUPPPORT

COMMUNITY FIRST CHOICE OPTION

(1)A State may provide through a State plan amendment for the provision of medical assistance for home and community-based attendant services and supports for individuals who are eligible for medical assistance under the State plan whose income does not exceed 150 percent of the poverty line (as defined in section 2110(c)(5)) or, if greater, the income level applicable for an individual who has been determined to require an institutional level of care to be eligible for nursing facility services under the State plan and with respect to whom there has been a determination that, but for the provision of such services, the individuals would require the level of care provided in a hospital, a nursing facility, an intermediate care facility for the mentally retarded, or an institution for mental diseases, the cost of which could be reimbursed under the State plan, but only if the individual chooses to receive such home and community-based attendant services and supports, and only if the State meets the following requirements:

(A) AVAILABILITY.—The State shall make available home and community-based attendant services and supports

to eligible individuals, as needed, to assist in accomplishing activities of daily living, instrumental activities of daily living, and health-related tasks through hands-on assistance, supervision, or cueing—

(i) under a person-centered plan of services and supports that is based on an assessment of functional need and that is agreed to in writing by the individual or, as appropriate, the individual's representative;

(ii) in a home or community setting, which does not include a nursing facility, institution for mental diseases, or an intermediate care facility for the mentally retarded;

(iii) under an agency-provider model or other model (as defined in paragraph (6) (C)); and

(iv) the furnishing of which —

(I) is selected, managed, and dismissed by the individual, or, as appropriate, with assistance from the individual's representative;

(II) is controlled, to the maximum extent possible, by the individual or where appropriate, the individual's representative, regardless of who may act as the employer of record; and

(III) provided by an individual who is qualified to provide such services, including family members (as defined by the Secretary).

(B) **INCLUDED SERVICES AND SUPPORTS.** — In addition to assistance in accomplishing activities of daily living, instrumental activities of daily living, and health related tasks, the home and community-based attendant services

and supports made available include —

(i) the acquisition, maintenance, and enhancement of skills necessary for the individual to accomplish activities of daily living, instrumental activities of daily living, and health related tasks;

(ii) back-up systems or mechanisms (such as the use of beepers or other electronic devices) to ensure continuity of services and supports; and

(iii) voluntary training on how to select, manage, and dismiss attendants.

(D) **PERMISSIBLE SERVICES AND SUPPORTS.** — The home and community-based attendant services and supports may include —

(i) expenditures for transition costs such as rent and utility deposits, first month's rent and utilities, bedding, basic kitchen supplies, and other necessities required for an individual to make the transition from a nursing facility, institution for mental diseases, or intermediate care facility for the mentally retarded to a community-based home setting where the individual resides; and

(ii) expenditures relating to a need identified in an individual's person-centered plan of services that increase independence or substitute for human assistance, to the extent that expenditures would otherwise be made for the human assistance.

(2) **INCREASED FEDERAL FINANCIAL PARTICIPATION.** (W)ith respect to amounts expended by the State to provide medical assistance under the State plan for home and community based attendant services and supports to eligible individuals in accordance with this subsection during a fiscal year quarter occurring during the period described in paragraph (1), the Federal medical assistance percentage applicable to the State (as determined under section 1905(b)) shall be increased by 6 percentage points.

WHAT THIS MEANS

Long term care is covered.

REMOVAL OF BARRIERS TO PROVIDING HOME AND COMMUNITY BASED SERVICES.

(a) OVERSIGHT AND ASSESSMENT OF THE ADMINISTRATION OF HOME AND COMMUNITY-BASED SERVICES.—The Secretary of Health and Human Services shall promulgate regulations to ensure that all States develop service systems that are designed to—

(1) allocate resources for services in a manner that is responsive[14] to the changing needs and choices of beneficiaries receiving non-institutionally-based long-term services and supports (including such services and supports that are provided under programs other the State Medicaid program), and that provides strategies for beneficiaries receiving such services to maximize their independence, including through the use of client employed providers;

(2) provide the support and coordination needed for a beneficiary in need of such services (and their family caregivers or representative, if applicable) to design an individualized, self directed, community-supported life.

WHAT THIS MEANS

It is easier to get home health and community care.

PRESCRIPTION DRUG REBATES

(a) INCREASE IN MINIMUM REBATE PERCENTAGE FOR SINGLE SOURCE DRUGS AND INNOVATOR MULTIPLE SOURCE DRUGS.(1)(B) (iii) MINIMUM REBATE PERCENTAGE FOR CERTAIN

DRUGS.(I) In the case of a single[15]source drug or an innovator multiple source drug), the minimum rebate percentage for rebate periods 17.1 percent.

(c) EXTENSION OF PRESCRIPTION DRUG DISCOUNTS TO ENROLLEES OF MEDICAID MANAGED CARE ORGANIZATIONS. (I) Covered outpatient drugs dispensed to individuals eligible for medical assistance who are enrolled with the entity shall be subject to the same rebate required by the agreement entered into under section 1927 as the State is subject to and that the State shall collect such rebates from manufacturers, (II) capitation rates paid to the entity shall be based on actual cost experience related to rebates and subject to the Federal regulations requiring actuarially sound rates, and (III) the entity shall report to the State, on such timely and periodic basis as specified by the Secretary in order to include in the information submitted by the State to a manufacturer and the Secretary under section 1927(b)(2)(A), information on the total number of units of each dosage form and strength and package size by

National Drug Code of each covered outpatient drug dispensed to individuals eligible for medical assistance who are enrolled with the entity and for which the entity is responsible for coverage of such drug under this subsection (other than covered outpatient drugs that under subsection (j)(1) of section 1927 are not subject to the requirements of that section) and such other data as the Secretary determines necessary to carry out this subsection.

(7) NON-EXCLUDABLE DRUGS.—The following drugs or classes of drugs, or their medical uses, shall not be excluded from coverage:

(A) Agents when used to promote smoking cessation, including agents approved by the Food and Drug Administration under the over-the-counter monograph process for purposes of promoting, and when used to promote, tobacco cessation. (B) Barbiturates. (C) Benzodiazepines.".

PROVIDING ADEQUATE PHARMACY REIMBURSEMENT

Any other discounts, rebates, payments, or other financial transactions that are received by, paid by, or passed through to, retail community pharmacies shall be included in the average manufacturer price for a covered[16] outpatient drug.

WHAT THIS MEANS

Reimbursement for prescription drugs must be adequate.

STATE OPTION TO PROVIDE HEALTH HOMES FOR ENROLLEES WITH CHRONIC CONDITIONS

A State shall provide a designated provider[17], a team of health care professionals operating with such a provider, or a health team with payments for the provision of health home services to each eligible individual with chronic conditions that selects such provider, team of health care professionals, or health team as the individual's health home. The term 'chronic condition' shall include, but is not limited to, the following: (A) A mental health condition.

(B) Substance use disorder. (C) Asthma. (D) Diabetes. (E) Heart disease. (F) Being overweight, as evidenced by having a Body Mass Index (BMI) over 25.

(B) SERVICES DESCRIBED.—The services described in this subparagraph are—(i) comprehensive care management;

(ii) care coordination and health promotion; (iii) comprehensive transitional care, including appropriate follow-up, from inpatient to other settings; (iv) patient and family support (including authorized representatives); (v) referral to community and social support services, if relevant; and (vi) use of health information technology to link services, as feasible and appropriate.

(6) **TEAM OF HEALTH CARE PROFESSIONALS.**—The term 'team of health care professionals' means a team of health professionals (as described in the State plan amendment) that may—

(A) include physicians and other professionals, such as a nurse care coordinator, nutritionist, social worker, behavioral health professional, or any professionals deemed appropriate by the State; and

DENTAL BENEFITS

(ii) OFFERING OF STAND-ALONE DENTAL BENEFITS. Each Exchange within a State shall allow an issuer of a plan that only provides limited scope dental benefits meeting the requirements of section 9832(c)(2) (A) of the Internal Revenue Code of 1986 to offer the plan through the Exchange (either separately or in conjunction with a qualified health plan) if the plan provides pediatric dental benefits meeting the requirements of section 1302(b) (1) (J)).

WHAT THIS MEANS

Dental benefits must be covered.

ADDITIONAL REQUIRED BENEFITS

(3) RULES RELATING TO ADDITIONAL REQUIRED BENEFITS.
(B) STATES MAY REQUIRE ADDITIONAL BENEFITS.
(i) IN GENERAL.—Subject to the requirements of clause (ii), a State may require that a qualified health plan offered in such State offer benefits in addition to the essential health benefits.
(ii) STATE MUST ASSUME COST. A State shall make payments—
(I) to an individual enrolled in a qualified health plan offered in such State; or
(II) on behalf of an individual described in sub clause (I) directly to the qualified health plan in which such individual is enrolled;
to defray the cost of any additional benefits.

WHAT THIS MEANS

States may provide additional coverage.

CONSUMER CHOICE

(a) CHOICE.—(1) QUALIFIED INDIVIDUALS A qualified individual may enroll in any qualified health plan available to such individual and for which such individual[18]is eligible.

(2) QUALIFIED EMPLOYERS.(A) EMPLOYER MAY SPECIFY LEVEL.—A qualified employer may provide support for coverage of employees under a qualified health plan by selecting any level of coverage under section 1302(d) to be made available to employees through an Exchange.

(B) EMPLOYEE MAY CHOOSE PLANS WITHIN A LEVEL. Each employee of a qualified employer that elects a level of coverage under subparagraph (A) may choose to enroll in a qualified health plan that offers coverage at that level.

(b) PAYMENT OF PREMIUMS BY QUALIFIED INDIVIDUALS.—A qualified individual enrolled in any qualified health plan may pay any applicable premium owed by such individual to the health insurance issuer issuing such qualified health plan.

(A) CHOICE TO ENROLL OR NOT TO ENROLL. — Nothing in this title shall be construed to restrict the choice of a qualified individual to enroll or not to enroll in a qualified health plan or to participate in an Exchange.

(B) PROHIBITION AGAINST COMPELLED ENROLLMENT. Nothing in this title shall be construed to compel an individual to enroll in a qualified health plan or to participate in an Exchange.

(C) INDIVIDUALS ALLOWED TO ENROLL IN ANY PLAN. A qualified individual may enroll in any qualified health plan, except that in the case of a catastrophic plan described in section 1302(e), a qualified individual may enroll

in the plan only if the individual is eligible to enroll in the plan under section 1302(e) (2).

WHAT THIS MEANS

Consumers may choose whether or not to participate in any specific plan...

LIFETIME OR ANNUAL LIMITS

IN GENERAL. — A group health plan and a health insurance issuer offering group or individual health insurance coverage may not establish— (A) lifetime limits on the dollar value of benefits for any participant or beneficiary; or (B) except as provided in paragraph (2), annual limits on the dollar value of benefits for any participant or beneficiary. [19]

WHAT THIS MEANS

There are no lifetime limits on the dollar value of benefits for any participant or beneficiary; or annual limits on the dollar value of benefits for any participant or beneficiary. [20]

PROHIBITION ON RESCISSIONS

A group health plan and a health insurance issuer offering group or individual health insurance coverage shall not rescind such plan or coverage with respect to an enrollee once the enrollee is covered under such plan or coverage involved, except that this section shall not apply to a covered individual who has performed an act or practice that constitutes fraud or makes an intentional misrepresentation of material fact as prohibited by the terms of the plan or coverage. Such plan or coverage may not be cancelled except with prior notice to the enrollee.[21]

WHAT THIS MEANS

Plan or coverage may not be cancelled.

CONSUMER OPERATED PLANS

Create four benefit categories of plans plus a separate catastrophic plan to be offered through the Exchange, and in the individual and small group markets: Bronze plan represents minimum creditable coverage and provides the essential health benefits, cover 60% of the benefit costs of the plan, with an out-of-pocket limit equal to the Health Savings Account (HSA) current law limit ($5,950 for individuals and $11,900 for families in 2010);

- Silver plan provides the essential health benefits, covers 70% of the benefit costs of the plan, with the HSA out-of-pocket limits;
- Gold plan provides the essential health benefits, covers 80% of the benefit costs of the plan, with the HSA out-of-pocket limits;
- Platinum plan provides the essential health benefits, covers 90% of the benefit costs of the plan, with the HSA out-of-pocket limits;
- Catastrophic plan available to those up to age 30 or to those who are exempt from the mandate to purchase coverage and provides catastrophic coverage only with the coverage level set at the HSA current law levels except that prevention benefits and coverage for three primary care visits would be exempt from the deductible. This plan is only available in the individual market.

Reduce the out-of-pocket limits for those with incomes up to 400% FPL[22] to the following levels:

- 100-200% FPL: one-third of the HSA limits ($1,983/individual and $3,967/family);

- 200-300% FPL: one-half of the HSA limits ($2,975/individual and $5,950/family);
- 300-400% FPL: two-thirds of the HSA limits ($3,987/individual and $7,973/family).

Require qualified health plans participating in the Exchange to meet marketing requirements, have adequate provider networks, contract with essential community providers, contract with navigators to conduct outreach and enrollment assistance, be accredited with respect to performance on quality measures, use a uniform enrollment form and standard format to present plan information.

Require qualified health plans to report information on claims payment policies, enrollment, disenrollment, number of claims denied, cost-sharing requirements, out-of-network policies, and enrollee rights in plain language.

Require the Exchanges to maintain a call center for customer service, and establish procedures for enrolling individuals and businesses and for determining eligibility for tax credits. Require states to develop a single form for applying for state health subsidy programs that can be filed online, in person, by mail or by phone.

Permit states the option to create a Basic Health Plan for uninsured individuals with incomes between 133-200% FPL who would otherwise be eligible to receive premium subsidies in the Exchange. States opting to provide this coverage will contract with one or more standard plans to provide at least the essential health benefits and must ensure that eligible individuals do not pay more in premiums than they would have paid in the Exchange and that the cost-sharing requirements do not exceed those of the platinum plan for enrollees with income less than 150% FPL or the gold plan for all other enrollees. States will receive 95% of the funds that would have been paid as federal premium and cost-sharing subsidies for eligible individuals to establish the Basic Health Plan. Individuals with incomes between 133-200% FPL in states creating Basic Health Plans will not be eligible for subsidies in the Exchanges.

WHAT THIS MEANS

Require qualified health plans participating in the Exchange to provide essential benefits required by OBAMACARE plus a separate catastrophic plan

ENSURING THE QUALITY OF CARE

(a) QUALITY REPORTING. — (1) (b) WELLNESS AND PREVENTION PROGRAMS. Wellness and health promotion activities may include personalized wellness and prevention services, which are coordinated, maintained or delivered by a health care provider, a wellness and prevention plan manager, or a health, wellness or prevention services organization that conducts health risk assessments or offers ongoing face-to-face, telephonic or web-based intervention efforts for each of the program's participants, and which may include the following wellness and prevention efforts:[23]

(1) Smoking cessation. (2) Weight management. (3) Stress management. (4) Physical fitness. (5) Nutrition. (6) Heart disease prevention. (7) Healthy lifestyle support. (8) Diabetes prevention.

WHAT THIS MEANS

Wellness and health promotion activities may include personalized wellness and prevention services, (1) Smoking cessation. (2) Weight management. (3) Stress management. (4) Physical fitness. (5) Nutrition. (6) Heart disease prevention. (7) Healthy lifestyle support. (8) Diabetes prevention.

APPEALS PROCESS

(a) INTERNAL CLAIMS APPEALS. — [24]

(1) A group health plan and a health insurance issuer offering group or individual health insurance coverage shall implement an effective appeals process for appeals of coverage determinations and claims, under which the plan or issuer shall, at a minimum —

(A) Have in effect an internal claims appeal process;

(B) Provide notice to enrollees, in a culturally and linguistically appropriate manner, of available internal and external appeals processes, and the availability of any applicable office of health insurance consumer assistance or ombudsman established under section 2793 to assist such enrollees with the appeals processes; and

(C) Allow an enrollee to review their file, to present evidence and testimony as part of the appeals process, and to receive continued coverage pending the outcome of the appeals process.

(b) EXTERNAL REVIEW.—A group health plan and a health insurance issuer offering group or individual health insurance coverage—
(1) Shall comply with the applicable State external review process for such plans and issuers that, at a minimum, includes the consumer protections set forth in the Uniform External Review Model Act promulgated by the National Association of Insurance Commissioners and is binding on such plans; or
(2) Shall implement an effective external review process that meets minimum standards established by the Secretary through guidance and that is similar to the process described under paragraph (1)—

WHAT THIS MEANS

Patients have the right to appeal decisions by insurers.

PREEXISTING CONDITION.

(A) Provides[25] to all eligible individuals health insurance coverage that does not impose any preexisting condition exclusion with respect to such coverage;
(d) ELIGIBLE INDIVIDUAL.—An individual shall be deemed to be an eligible individual if such individual—
(1) Is a citizen or national of the United States or is lawfully present in the United States (as determined in accordance with section 1411);
(3) Has a pre-existing condition, as determined in a manner consistent with guidance issued by the Secretary.

WHAT THIS MEANS

Pre-existing conditions are covered.

GUARANTEED AVAILABILITY OF COVERAGE

Subject to subsections (b) through (e), each health insurance issuer that offers health insurance coverage in the individual or group market in a State must accept every employer and individual in the State that applies for such coverage.[26]

WHAT THIS MEANS

Group insurance must cover every employee.

GUARANTEED RENEWABILITY OF COVERAGE

(a) Except as provided in this section, if a health insurance issuer offers health insurance coverage in the individual or group market, the issuer must renew or continue in force such coverage at the option of the plan sponsor or the individual, as applicable.[27]

WHAT THIS MEANS

Coverage must be renewed.

HEALTH STATUS

(a) A group health plan and a health insurance issuer offering group or individual health insurance coverage may[28] not establish rules for eligibility (including continued eligibility) of any individual to enroll under the terms of the plan or coverage based on any of the following health status-related factors in relation to the individual or a dependent of the individual:

(1) Health status. (2) Medical condition (including both physical and mental illnesses). (3) Claims experience. (4) Receipt of health care. (5) Medical history. (6) Genetic information. (7) Evidence of insurability (including conditions arising out of acts of domestic violence). (8) Disability. (9) Any other health status-related factor determined appropriate by the Secretary.

WHAT THIS MEANS

Health status of a person is not to be considered when issuing coverage.

PROGRAMS OF HEALTH PROMOTION OR DISEASE PREVENTION.

A program of health promotion or disease prevention (referred to in this subsection as a 'wellness program') shall be a program offered by an employer that is designed to promote health or prevent disease that meets the applicable requirements of this subsection.

WHAT THIS MEANS

Health promotion or disease prevention shall be a program offered by an employer that is designed to promote health or prevent disease.

OBAMACARE-TRUMPCARE

PROHIBITION ON EXCESSIVE WAITING PERIODS

A group health plan and a[29]health insurance issuer offering group health insurance coverage shall not apply any waiting period that exceeds 90 days.

WHAT THIS MEANS

Group plans cannot have more than 90 days of waiting.

CHOICE OF HEALTH CARE PROFESSIONAL

If a group health plan, or a health insurance issuer offering group or individual health insurance coverage, requires or provides for designation by a participant, beneficiary, or enrollee of a participating primary care provider, then the plan or issuer shall permit each participant, beneficiary, and enrollee to designate any participating primary care provider who is available to accept such individual.

WHAT THIS MEANS

One may choose the professionals who may provide care.

ESSENTIAL BENEFITS

Create an essential health benefits package that provides a comprehensive set of services, covers at least 60% of the actuarial value of the covered benefits, limits annual cost-sharing to the current law HSA limits ($5,950/individual and $11,900/family in 2010), and is not more extensive than the typical employer plan. Require all qualified health benefits plans, including those offered through the Exchanges and those offered in the individual and small group markets outside the Exchanges, except grandfathered individual and employer-sponsored plans, to offer at least the essential health benefits package. Prohibit abortion coverage from being required as part of the essential health benefits package.

WHAT THIS MEANS

Plans must provide OBAMACARE benefits.

CHANGES TO PRIVATE INSURANCE

Establish a temporary national high-risk pool to provide health coverage to individuals with pre-existing medical conditions. U.S. citizens and legal immigrants who have a pre-existing medical condition and who have been uninsured for at least six months will be eligible to enroll in the high-risk pool and receive subsidized premiums. Premiums for the pool will be established for a standard population and may vary by no more than 4 to 1 due to age; maximum cost-sharing will be limited to the current law HSA limit ($5,950/individual and $11,900/family in 2010).

Require health plans to report the proportion of premium dollars spent on clinical services, quality, and other costs and provide rebates to consumers for the amount of the premium spent on clinical services and quality that is less than 85% for plans in the large group market and 80% for plans in the individual and small group markets.

Establish a process for reviewing increases in health plan premiums and require plans to justify increases. Require states to report on trends in premium increases and recommend whether certain plan should be excluded from the Exchange based on unjustified premium increases. Provide grants to states to support efforts to review and approve premium increases.

WHAT THIS MEANS

Insurance companies must provide OBAMACARE benefits.

DEPENDENT COVERAGE

Provide dependent coverage for children up to age 26 for all individual and group policies.

WHAT THIS MEANS

Children up to age 26 must be covered under plans.

INSURANCE MARKETS

Prohibit individual and group health plans from placing lifetime limits on the dollar value of coverage and prohibit insurers from rescinding coverage except in cases of fraud. Prohibit pre-existing condition exclusions for children. Prohibit individual and group health plans from placing annual limits on the dollar value of coverage. Prior to January 2014, plans may only impose annual limits on coverage as determined by the Secretary.

Grandfather existing individual and group plans with respect to new benefit standards, but require these grandfathered plans to extend dependent coverage to adult children up to age 26 and prohibit rescissions of coverage. Require grandfathered group plans to eliminate lifetime limits on coverage and beginning in 2014, eliminate annual limits on coverage. Prior to 2014, grandfathered group plans may only impose annual limits as determined by the Secretary. Require grandfathered group plans to eliminate pre-existing condition exclusions for children within six months of enactment and by 2014 for adults, and eliminate waiting periods for coverage of greater than 90 days by 2014.

Impose the same insurance market regulations relating to guarantee issue, premium rating, and prohibitions on pre-existing condition exclusions in the individual market, in the Exchange, and in the small group market.

Require all new policies (except stand-alone dental, vision, and long-term care insurance plans), including those offered through the Exchanges and those offered outside of the Exchanges, to comply with one of the four benefit categories. Existing individual and employer-sponsored plans do not have to meet the new benefit standards.

Limit deductibles for health plans in the small group market to $2,000 for individuals and $4,000 for families unless contributions are offered that offset deductible amounts above these limits. This deductible limit will not affect the actuarial value of any plans. Limit any waiting periods for coverage to 90 days.

WHAT THIS MEANS

Insurance markets must provide OBAMACARE benefits.

HEALTHCARE CHOICE COMPACTS

Permit states to form health care choice compacts and allow insurers to sell policies in any state participating in the compact. Insurers selling policies through a compact would only be subject to the laws and regulations of the state where the policy is written or issued, except for rules pertaining to market conduct, unfair trade practices, network adequacy, and consumer protections. Compacts may only be approved if it is determined that the compact will provide coverage that is at least as comprehensive and affordable as coverage provided through the state Exchanges

WHAT THIS MEANS

Health care choice compacts must provide OBAMACARE benefits.

ROLE OF STATES

States who participate must create an American Health Benefit Exchange and a Small Business Health Options Program (SHOP) Exchange for individuals and small businesses and provide oversight of health plans with regard to the new insurance market regulations, consumer protections, rate reviews, solvency, reserve fund requirements, premium taxes, and to define rating areas.

They must enroll newly eligible Medicaid beneficiaries into the Medicaid program no later than January 2014 (states have the option to expand enrollment beginning in 2011), coordinate enrollment with the new Exchanges, and implement other specified changes to the Medicaid program. Maintain current Medicaid and CHIP eligibility levels for children until 2019 and maintain current Medicaid eligibility levels for adults until the Exchange is fully operational. A state will be exempt from the maintenance of effort requirement for non-disabled adults with incomes above 133% FPL for any year from January 2011 through December 31, 2013 if the state certifies that it is experiencing a budget deficit or will experience a deficit in the following year.

They must establish an office of health insurance consumer assistance or an ombudsman program to serve as an advocate for people with private coverage in the individual and small group markets. (Federal grants available beginning fiscal year 2010)

States may create a Basic Health Plan for uninsured individuals with incomes between 133% and 200% FPL in lieu of these individuals receiving premium subsidies to purchase coverage in the Exchanges. Permit states to obtain a five-year waiver of certain new health insurance requirements if the state can demonstrate that it provides health coverage to all residents that is at least as comprehensive as the coverage required under an Exchange plan and that the state plan does not increase the federal budget deficit.

WHAT THIS MEANS

States who participate must create an American Health Benefit Exchange and a Small Business Health Options Program (SHOP) Exchange for individuals and small Business and must provide OBAMACARE benefits. They may expand Medicaid program to cover all.

DUAL ELIGIBLES

Improve care coordination for dual eligible's by creating a new office within the Centers for Medicare and Medicaid services, the Federal Coordinated Health Care Office, to more effectively integrate Medicare and Medicaid benefits and improve coordination between the federal government and states in order to improve access to and quality of care and services for dual eligible's.

WHAT THIS MEANS

Medicare and Medicaid benefits to those who qualify for both are to be coordinated.

FRAUD AND ABUSE

(5) PROTECTIONS AGAINST FRAUD AND ABUSE.—With respect to activities carried out under this title, the Secretary shall provide for the efficient and non-discriminatory administration of Exchange activities and implement any measure or procedure that—

(A) the Secretary determines is appropriate to reduce fraud and abuse in the administration of this title; and

(B) the Secretary has authority to implement under this title or any other Act.

(6) APPLICATION OF THE FALSE CLAIMS ACT.—

(A) IN GENERAL.—Payments made by, through, or in connection with an Exchange are subject to the False Claims Act (31 U.S.C. 3729 et seq.) if those payments include any Federal funds. Compliance with the requirements of this Act concerning eligibility for a health insurance issuer to participate in the Exchange shall be a material condition of an issuer's entitlement to receive payments, including payments of premium tax credits and cost-sharing reductions, through the Exchange.

(B) DAMAGES.—Notwithstanding paragraph (1) of section 3729(a) of title 31, United States Code, and subject to paragraph (2) of such section, the civil penalty assessed under the False Claims Act on any person found liable under such Act as described in subparagraph (A) shall be increased by not less than 3 times and not more than 6 times the amount of damages which the Government sustains because of the act of that person..

(4)(A) The court shall dismiss an action or claim under this section, unless opposed by the Government, if substantially the same allegations or transactions as alleged in the action or claim were publicly disclosed —

(i) in a Federal criminal, civil, or administrative hearing in which the Government or its agent is a party;

(ii) in a congressional, Government Accountability Office, or other Federal report, hearing, audit, or investigation;

or

(iii) from the news media, unless the action is brought by the Attorney General or the person bringing the action is an original source of the information.

(B) For purposes of this paragraph, "original source" means an individual who either (i) prior to a public disclosure under subsection (e) (4) (a), has voluntarily disclosed to the Government the information on which allegations or transactions in a claim are based, or (2) who has knowledge that is independent of and materially adds to the publicly disclosed allegations to the Government before filing an action under this section.

STATE FLEXIBILITY TO ESTABLISH ALTERNATIVE PROGRAMS

(a) ESTABLISHMENT OF PROGRAM.

(1) IN GENERAL. — The Secretary shall establish a basic[30] health program meeting the requirements of this section under which a State may enter into contracts to offer 1 or more standard health plans providing at least the essential health benefits described in section 1302(b) to eligible individuals in lieu of offering such individuals coverage through an Exchange.

(b) STANDARD HEALTH PLAN. — In this section, the term "standard heath plan" means a health benefits plan that the State contracts with under this section

(1) Under which the only individuals eligible to enroll are eligible individuals;

(2) That provides at least the essential health benefits described in section 1302(b); and

(3) in the case of a plan that provides health insurance coverage offered by a health insurance issuer, that has a medical loss ratio of at least 85 percent.

(c) CONTRACTING PROCESS.—

(2) SPECIFIC ITEMS TO BE CONSIDERED.—A State shall, as part of its competitive process under paragraph (1), include at least the following:

(A) INNOVATION.—Negotiation with offerors of a standard health plan for the inclusion of innovative features in the plan, including— (i) care coordination and care management for enrollees, especially for those with chronic health conditions; (ii) incentives for use of preventive services; and (iii) the establishment of relationships between providers and patients that maximize patient involvement in health care decision-making, including providing incentives for appropriate utilization under the plan.

(B) HEALTH AND RESOURCE DIFFERENCES.—Consideration of, and the making of suitable allowances for, differences in health care needs of enrollees and differences in local availability of, and access to, health care providers. Nothing in this subparagraph shall be construed as allowing discrimination on the basis of pre-existing conditions or other health status-related factors.

(C) MANAGED CARE.—Contracting with managed care systems, or with systems that offer as many of the attributes of managed care as are feasible in the local health care market.

(D) PERFORMANCE MEASURES.—Establishing specific performance measures and standards for issuers of standard health plans that focus on quality of care and improved health outcomes, requiring such plans to report to the State with respect to the measures and standards, and making the performance and quality information available to enrollees in a useful form.

(3) ENHANCED AVAILABILITY.—

(A) MULTIPLE PLANS.—A State shall, to the maximum extent feasible, seek to make multiple standard health plans available to eligible individuals within a State to ensure individuals have a choice of such plans.

(B) REGIONAL COMPACTS.—A State may negotiate a regional compact with other States to include coverage of eligible individuals in all such States in agreements with issuers of standard health plans.

WHAT THIS MEANS

States may establish alternative programs.

PREMIUM TAX CREDITS AND COSTSHARING REDUCTIONS

REFUNDABLE CREDIT FOR COVERAGE UNDER A QUALIFIED HEALTH PLAN.

(a) IN GENERAL. — In the case of an applicable taxpayer, there shall be allowed as a credit against the tax imposed by this subtitle for any taxable year an amount equal to the premium assistance credit amount of the taxpayer for the taxable year.[31]

(b) PREMIUM ASSISTANCE CREDIT AMOUNT. — For purposes of this section (1) The term 'premium assistance credit amount' means, with respect to any taxable year, the sum of the premium assistance amounts determined under paragraph (2) with respect to all coverage months of the taxpayer occurring during the taxable year.

(2) PREMIUM ASSISTANCE AMOUNT. — The premium assistance amount determined under this subsection with respect to any coverage month is the amount equal to the lesser of (A) the monthly premiums for such month for 1 or more qualified health plans offered in the individual market within a State which cover the taxpayer, the taxpayer's spouse, or any dependent (as defined in section 152) of the taxpayer and which were enrolled in through an Exchange established by the State under 1311 of the Patient Protection and Affordable Care Act, or (B) the excess (if any) of (i) the adjusted monthly premium for such month for the applicable second lowest cost silver plan with respect to the taxpayer, over (ii) an amount equal to 1/12 of the product of the applicable percentage and the taxpayer's household income for the taxable year.

(3) (A) APPLICABLE PERCENTAGE. (i) IN GENERAL Except as provided in clause (ii), the applicable percentage for any taxable year shall be the percentage such that the applicable percentage for any taxpayer whose household income is within an income tier specified in the following table shall increase, on a sliding scale in a linear manner, from the initial premium percentage to the final premium percentage specified in such table for such income tier:

In the case of household income (expressed as a percent of poverty line) within the following income tier:

The initial premium percentage is The final premium percentage is
Up to 133% 2.0% 2.0%
    133% up to 150% 3.0% 4.0%
    150% up to 200% 4.0% 6.3%

200% up to 250% 6.3% 8.05%
250% up to 300% 8.05% 9.5%
300% up to 400% 9.5% 9.5%

ADDITIONAL BENEFITS

(D) ADDITIONAL BENEFITS. If (i) a qualified health plan under section 1302(b)(5) of the Patient Protection and Affordable Care Act offers benefits in addition to the essential health benefits required to be provided by the plan, or (ii) a State requires a qualified health plan under section 1311(d)(3)(B) of such Act to cover benefits in addition to the essential health benefits required to be provided by the plan, the portion of the premium for the plan properly allocable (under rules prescribed by the Secretary of Health and Human Services) to such additional benefits shall not be taken into account in determining either the monthly premium or the adjusted monthly premium under paragraph (2).

WHAT THIS MEANS

Plans may offer additional benefits.

SPECIAL RULE FOR PEDIATRIC DENTAL COVERAGE

(E) For purposes of determining the amount of any monthly[32] premium, if an individual enrolls in both a qualified health plan and a plan described in section 1311(d)(2)(B)(ii)(I) of the Patient Protection and Affordable Care Act for any plan year, the portion of the premium for the plan described in such section that (under regulations prescribed by the Secretary) is properly allocable to pediatric dental benefits which are included in the essential health benefits required to be provided by a qualified health plan under section 1302(b) (1) (J) of such Act shall be treated as a premium payable for a qualified health plan.

RELIGIOUS EXEMPTIONS

(A) RELIGIOUS CONSCIENCE EXEMPTION. Such term shall not include any individual for any month if such individual has in effect an exemption under section 1311(d) (4)(H) of the Patient Protection and Affordable Care Act which certifies that such individual is —

(i) a member of a recognized religious sect or division thereof which is described in section 1402(g)(1), and (ii) an adherent of established tenets or teachings of such sector division as described in such section.

HEALTH CARE SHARING MINISTRY

(ii) The term 'health care sharing ministry' means an organization—

(I) which is described in section 501(c) (3) and is exempt from taxation under section 501(a),

(II) members of which share a common set of ethical or religious beliefs and share medical expenses among members in accordance with those beliefs and without regard to the State in which a member resides or is employed,

(III) members of which retain membership even after they develop a medical condition,

(IV) which (or a predecessor of which) has been in existence at all times since December 31, 1999, and medical expenses of its members have been shared continuously and without interruption since at least December 31, 1999.

WHAT THIS MEANS

Groups can be made of those with similar ethical or religious beliefs.

INDIVIDUALS WHO CANNOT AFFORD COVERAGE

(A) IN GENERAL.—Any applicable individual for any month if the applicable individual's required contribution (determined on an annual basis) for coverage for the month exceeds 8 percent of such individual's household income for the taxable year described in section 1412(b)(1)(B) of the Patient Protection and Affordable Care Act. For purposes of applying this subparagraph, the taxpayer's household income shall be increased by any exclusion from gross.

WHAT THIS MEANS

People who cannot afford coverage shall be provided government assistance.

FREEDOM NOT TO PARTICIPATE IN FEDERAL HEALTH INSURANCE PROGRAMS

No individual, company, business, nonprofit entity,[33] or health insurance issuer offering group or individual health insurance coverage shall be required to participate in any Federal health insurance program created under this Act (or any amendments made by this Act), or in any Federal health insurance program expanded by this Act (or any such amendments), and there shall be no penalty or fine imposed upon any such issuer for choosing not to participate in such programs.

NONDISCRIMINATION

(a) IN GENERAL.—Except as otherwise provided for in this title (or an amendment made by this title), an individual shall not, on[34] the ground prohibited under title VI of the Civil Rights Act of 1964 (42 U.S.C. 2000d et seq.), title IX of the Education Amendments of 1972 (20 U.S.C. 1681 et seq.), the Age Discrimination Act of 1975(42 U.S.C. 6101 et seq.), or section 504 of the Rehabilitation Act of 1973 (29 U.S.C. 794), be excluded from participation in, be denied the benefits of, or be subjected to discrimination under, any health program or activity, any part of which is receiving Federal financial assistance, including credits, subsidies, or contracts of insurance, or under any program or activity that is administered by an Executive Agency or any entity established under this title (or amendments). The enforcement mechanisms provided for and available under such title VI, title IX, section 504, or such Age Discrimination Act shall apply for purposes of violations of this subsection.

PROTECTIONS FOR EMPLOYEES

SEC. 18C PROTECTIONS FOR EMPLOYEES

(a) PROHIBITION.—No employer[35] shall discharge or in any manner discriminate against any employee with respect to his or her compensation, terms, conditions, or other privileges of employment because the employee (or an individual acting at the request of the employee) has—

(1) received a credit under section 36B of the Internal Revenue Code of 1986 or a subsidy under section 1402 of this
Act;

(2) provided, caused to be provided, or is about to provide or cause to be provided to the employer, the Federal Government, or the attorney general of a State information relating to any violation of, or any act or omission the employee reasonably believes to be a violation of, any provision of this title (or an amendment made by this title);

(3) testified or is about to testify in a proceeding concerning such violation;

(4) assisted or participated, or is about to assist or participate, in such a proceeding; or

(5) objected to, or refused to participate in, any activity, policy, practice, or assigned task that the employee (or other

such person) reasonably believed to be in violation of any provision of this title (or amendment), or any order, rule, regulation, standard, or ban under this title (or amendment).

(b) **COMPLAINT PROCEDURE.**

(1) IN GENERAL. — An employee who believes that he or she has been discharged or otherwise discriminated against by any employer in violation of this section may seek relief in accordance with the procedures, notifications, burdens of proof, remedies, and statutes of limitation set forth in section 2087(b) of title 15, United States Code.

(2) NO LIMITATION ON RIGHTS. — Nothing in this section shall be deemed to diminish the rights, privileges, or remedies of any employee under any Federal or State law or under any collective bargaining agreement. The rights and remedies in this section may not be waived by any agreement, policy, form, or condition of employment.

WHAT THIS MEANS

Employees cannot be fired, demoted or punished for seeking coverage.

STATES MAY EXPAND ELIGIBILITY

(B) STATES MAY EXPAND ELIGIBILITY OR MOVE WAIVERED POPULATIONS INTO COVERAGE UNDER THE STATE PLAN. — With respect to any period applicable under paragraph (1), (2), or (3), a State that applies eligibility standards, methodologies, or procedures under the State plan under this title or under any waiver of the plan that are less restrictive than the eligibility standards, methodologies, or procedures, applied under the State plan or under a waiver of the plan on the date of enactment of the Patient Protection and Affordable Care Act, or that makes individuals who, on such date of enactment, are eligible for medical assistance under a waiver of the State plan, after such date of enactment eligible for medical assistance through a State plan amendment with an income eligibility level that is not less than the income eligibility level that applied under the waiver, or as a result of the application of sub clause (VIII) of section 1902(a) (10) (A) (i), shall not be considered to have in effect eligibility standards, methodologies, or procedures that are more restrictive than the standards, methodologies, or procedures in effect under the State plan or under a waiver of the plan on the date of enactment of the Patient Protection and Affordable Care Act for purposes of determining compliance with the requirements of paragraph (1), (2), or (3).

MEDICAID MINIMUM BENEFITS

(c) MEDICAID BENCHMARK BENEFITS MUST CONSIST OF AT LEAST MINIMUM ESSENTIAL COVERAGE.—Section 1937(b) of such Act (42 U.S.C. 1396u-7(b)) is amended—

(5) MINIMUM STANDARDS.—Effective January 1, 2014, any benchmark benefit package under paragraph (1) or benchmark equivalent coverage under paragraph (2) must provide at least essential health benefits as described in section 1302(b) of the Patient Protection and Affordable Care Act.

(6) MENTAL HEALTH SERVICES PARITY.

(A) IN GENERAL.—In the case of any benchmark benefit package under paragraph (1) or benchmark equivalent coverage under paragraph (2) that is offered by an entity that is not a Medicaid managed care organization and that provides both medical and surgical benefits and mental health or substance use disorder benefits, the entity shall ensure that the financial requirements and treatment limitations applicable to such mental health or substance use disorder benefits comply with the requirements of section 2705(a) of the Public Health Service Act in the same manner as such requirements apply to a group health plan.

WHAT THIS MEANS

Medicaid must provide the coverage required by Obamacare.

(B) be free standing, virtual, or based at a hospital, community health center, community mental health center, rural clinic, clinical practice or clinical group practice, academic health center, or any entity deemed appropriate by the State and approved by the Secretary.

HOW TRUMP CARE HURTS AMERICANS

The[36] House speaker, Paul Ryan, and other Republicans falsely accused Democrats of rushing the Affordable Care Act through Congress.

In a display of breathtaking hypocrisy, House Republicans — without holding any hearings or giving the Congressional Budget Office time to do an analysis — passed a bill that would strip at least 24 million Americans of health insurance.

Obamacare: The nonpartisan Congressional Budget Office (CBO) estimated that if the ACA continues to be the law of the land, the number of uninsured Americans - currently 28 million - would remain stable for the next decade.

Trumpcare: The CBO did not have time to predict the potential effects of the latest version of the American Health Care Act (AHCA). In an analysis of an earlier version of the bill, the office found that a total of 54 million could be uninsured by 2026 if the AHCA becomes law.

It's estimated that 22 million would lose medical insurance if Obamacare were repealed. Provisions of the law make care accessible to those who had previously been shut out. The uninsured rate has dropped by 5% since the programme began.

Obamacare: All Americans must have health insurance or pay a tax penalty.

Trumpcare: The AHCA repeals the mandate, but those who go without health insurance for more than 63 days must pay a 30 per cent surcharge on their insurance premiums for a year.

Obamacare: Companies with more than 50 employees are required to provide health insurance or pay a penalty.

Trumpcare: The AHCA repeals the employer mandate.

Obamacare: To pay for the new system, the ACA raised Medicare taxes on those with incomes above $250,000. It also imposed new taxes on makers of medical devices, health insurers, drug companies, investment income, tanning salons and high-end health insurance plans. The legislation gave some tax credits to middle-income earners to help them pay out-of-pocket health expenses.

Trumpcare: The AHCA repeals most Obamacare taxes.

Some of the more popular provisions include:

- Children can stay on their parent's health care plan until age 26
- No one can be denied insurance for a pre-existing medical condition

- Companies can no longer charge women more than men
- health care providers and pharmacy companies.

Obamacare: Mandates that all insurance plans cover certain health conditions and services, such as annual physical exams, prescription drug costs, mental health counseling and women's health services.

Trumpcare: Enables states to waive requirements set forth in the ACA.

Obamacare: Expanded Medicaid health insurance for low-income individuals.

Trumpcare: Cuts federal funding for Medicaid expansion starting in 2020.

Obamacare: Prevents health insurers from denying coverage or charging more to individuals who have pre-existing medical conditions, such as asthma or heart disease.

Trumpcare: Allows states to waive rules that currently stop insurers from charging new customers more because of their medical history. States can opt out of the ACA requirements if they set up high-risk insurance plans, known as high-risk pools, for individuals who cannot afford traditional insurance. A new amendment provides an extra $8 billion to subsidise the cost of insuring those with pre-existing conditions.

As the law has been implemented there have been certain sections that work better than others, and some that cause problems for consumers. The Obama administration and Democratic members of Congress have tried to push through fixes that they say would alleviate these problems; the Republicans say the flaws are evidence of a failed programme.

Pushed by President Trump to repeal the A.C.A., or Obamacare, so he could claim a legislative win, Mr. Ryan and his lieutenants browbeat and cajoled members of their caucus to pass the bill. Groups representing doctors, hospitals, nurses, older people and people with illnesses like cancer opposed the bill. Just 17 percent of Americans supported an earlier version of the measure, and Republicans have made the legislation only worse since that poll was conducted. Neither Mr. Trump nor Mr. Ryan seemed bothered by this overwhelming criticism of their Trumpcare bill, the American Health Care Act. They seemed concerned only about appeasing the House Freedom Caucus, the far-right flank of their party.

Mr. Trump in particular has been spreading misinformation and lies about health care, arguing that the legislation would lower costs while guaranteeing that people with pre-existing health conditions could get affordable health insurance. It would do the opposite. Here is what the bill actually does:

The bill would cut $880 billion over 10 years from Medicaid, the program that provides health care to about 74 million poor, disabled and elderly Americans. That's one-fourth of its budget. As a result, 14 million fewer people would have access to health care by 2026, according to a C.B.O. analysis of the earlier bill, which contained similar Medicaid provisions. The cuts would also hurt special education programs, which receive about $4 billion from Medicaid every year.

It would provide $300 billion less over 10 years to help people who do not get insurance through employers and have to buy their own policies. This would hurt lower-income and older people the hardest. For example, a 60-year-old living in Phoenix and earning $40,000 would have to pay an additional $12,370 a year to buy a policy, according to the Kaiser Family Foundation. Many people who find themselves in this situation would have no choice but to forgo insurance.

Republicans say the law imposes too many costs on business, with many describing it as a "job killer". However, since the implementation of Obamacare, jobs in the health care sector rose by 9%.

I. Executive Summary Of Rules By DEPARTMENT OF HEALTH

Affordable Health Benefit Exchanges, or "Exchanges" are competitive marketplaces through which qualified individuals and qualified employers can purchase health insurance coverage. Many individuals who enroll in qualified health plans (QHPs) through individual market Exchanges are eligible to receive advance payments of the premium tax credit to reduce their costs for health insurance premiums, and receive reductions in cost-sharing payments to reduce out-of-pocket expenses for healthcare services.

The stability and competitiveness of the Exchanges, as well as that of the individual and small group markets in general, have recently been threatened by issuer exits and increasing rates in many geographic areas. Some issuers have had difficulty attracting and retaining the healthy consumers necessary to provide for a stable risk pool that will support stable rates. In particular, some issuers have cited special enrollment periods and grace periods as potential sources of adverse selection that have contributed to this problem. Concerns over the risk pool have led some issuers to cease offering coverage on the Exchanges in particular States and counties, and other issuers have increased their rates.

A stabilized individual and small group insurance market will depend on greater choice to draw consumers to the market and vibrant competition to ensure consumers have access to competitively priced, affordable, and quality coverage. Higher rates, particularly for consumers who are not receiving advance payments of the premium tax credit (APTC) or claiming the premium tax credit, resulting from minimal choice and competition, can cause healthier individuals to drop out of the market, further damaging the risk pool and risking additional issuer attrition from the market. This final rule takes steps to provide needed flexibility to issuers to help attract healthy consumers to enroll in health insurance coverage, improve the risk pool and bring stability and certainty to the individual and small group markets, while increasing the options for patients and providers.

To improve the risk pool and promote stability in the individual insurance markets, we are taking several steps to increase the incentives for individuals to maintain enrollment in health coverage and decrease the incentives for individuals to enroll only after they discover they require medical services. First, we are changing the dates for open enrollment in the individual markets for the benefit year starting January 1, 2018, from November 1, 2017 through January 31, 2018 (the previously established open enrollment period for 2018), to extend from November 1 through December 15, 2017. This change requires individuals to enroll in coverage prior to the beginning of the year, unless eligible for a special enrollment period, and is consistent with the open enrollment period previously established for the benefit years starting January 1, 2019, and beyond. This change will improve individual market risk pools by reducing opportunities for adverse selection by those who learn they will need medical services in late December and January; and will encourage healthier individuals who might have previously enrolled in partial year coverage after December 15th to instead enroll in coverage for the full year.

Second, we are responding to concerns from issuers about potential misuse and abuse of special enrollment periods in the individual market Exchanges that enables individuals who are not entitled to special enrollment periods to enroll in coverage after they realize they will need medical services. We are increasing pre-enrollment verification of all applicable individual market special enrollment periods for all States served by the HealthCare.gov platform from 50 to 100 percent of new consumers who seek to enroll in Exchange coverage through these special enrollment periods. We are also making several additional changes to our regulations regarding special enrollment periods that we believe could improve the risk pool, improve market stability, promote continuous coverage, and increase options for patients.

Third, we are revising our interpretation of the Federal guaranteed availability requirement to allow issuers, subject to applicable State law, to apply a premium payment to an individual's past debt owed for coverage from the same issuer or a different issuer in the same controlled group within the prior 12 months before applying the payment toward a new enrollment. We believe this interpretation will have a positive impact on the risk pool by removing economic incentives individuals may have had to pay premiums only when they were in need of healthcare services, particularly toward the end of the benefit year. We also believe this policy is an important means of encouraging individuals to maintain continuous coverage throughout the year.

Fourth, we are finalizing an increase in the de minimis variation in the actuarial values (AVs) used to determine metal levels of coverage for the 2018 plan year and beyond. This change is intended to allow issuers greater flexibility in designing new plans and to provide additional options for issuers to keep cost sharing the same from year to year, while helping stabilize premiums for consumers.

We believe these changes are critical to improving the risk pool, and will together promote more competitive markets with increased choice for consumers.

We are also finalizing policies intended to affirm the traditional role of States in overseeing their health insurance markets while reducing the regulatory burden of participating in Exchanges for issuers. The modified approach we are finalizing for network adequacy, which includes deferring to States with sufficient network adequacy review (or relying on accreditation or an access plan), will not only lessen the regulatory burden on issuers, but also will recognize the primary role of States in regulating this area. We are also finalizing changes that will allow issuers to continue to use a write-in process to identify essential community providers (ECPs) who are not on the HHS list of available ECPs for the 2018 plan year; and will lower the ECP standard to 20 percent (rather than 30 percent) for the 2018 plan year, which we believe will make it easier for a QHP issuer to build provider networks that comply with the ECP standard.

Robust issuer participation in the individual and small group markets is critical for ensuring consumers have access to affordable, quality coverage, and have real choice in coverage. Continued uncertainty around the future of the markets and concerns regarding the risk pools are two of the primary reasons issuer participation in some areas around the country has been limited. The changes in this rule are intended to promote issuer participation in these markets and to address concerns raised by issuers, States, and consumers. We believe these changes will result in broader choices and more affordable coverage.

II. Background

A. Legislative and Regulatory Overview

The Patient Protection and Affordable Care Act (Pub. L. 111-148) was enacted on March 23, 2010. The Health Care and Education Reconciliation Act of 2010 (Pub. L. 111-152), which amended and revised several provisions of the Patient Protection and Affordable Care Act, was enacted on March 30, 2010. In this final rule, we refer to the two statutes collectively as the "Patient Protection and Affordable Care Act" or "PPACA."

The PPACA reorganizes, amends, and adds to the provisions of title XXVII of the Public Health Service Act (PHS Act) relating to group health plans and health insurance issuers in the group and individual markets.

Section 2702 of the PHS Act, as added by the PPACA, requires health insurance issuers that offer non- grandfathered health insurance coverage in the group or individual market in a State to offer coverage to and accept every employer and individual in the State that applies for such coverage, unless an exception applies.

Section 2703 of the PHS Act, as added by the PPACA, and sections 2712 and 2742 of the PHS Act, as added by the Health Insurance Portability and Accountability Act of 1996 (HIPAA),[37] require health insurance issuers that offer health insurance coverage in the group or individual market to renew or continue in force such coverage at the option of the plan sponsor or individual, unless an exception applies.

Section 1302(d) of the PPACA describes the various metal levels of coverage based on AV. Consistent with section 1302(d)(2)(A) of the PPACA,

AV is calculated based on the provision of essential health benefits (EHB) to a standard population. Section 1302(d)(3) of the PPACA directs the Secretary to develop guidelines that allow for de minimis variation in AV calculations. Section 2707(a) of the PHS Act directs health insurance issuers that offer non- grandfathered health insurance coverage in the individual or small group market to ensure that such coverage includes the EHB package, which includes the requirement to offer coverage at the metal levels of coverage described in section 1302(d) of the PPACA.

Section 1311(c)(1)(B) of the PPACA requires the Secretary to establish minimum QHP certification criteria for provider network adequacy that a health plan must meet.

Section 1311(c)(1)(C) of the PPACA requires the Secretary to establish minimum QHP certification criteria for the inclusion of essential community providers.

Section 1311(c)(6)(B) of the PPACA states that the Secretary is to set annual open enrollment periods for Exchanges for calendar years after the initial enrollment period.

Section 1311(c)(6)(C) of the PPACA states that the Secretary is to provide for special enrollment periods specified in section 9801 of the Internal Revenue Code of 1986 (the Code) and other special enrollment periods under circumstances similar to such periods under part D of title XVIII of the Social Security Act (the Act) for the Exchanges.

Section 1321(a) of the PPACA provides broad authority for the Secretary to establish standards and regulations to implement the statutory requirements related to Exchanges, QHPs and other components of title I of the PPACA.

1. Market Rules

A proposed rule relating to the 2014 Health Insurance Market Rules was published in the November 26, 2012 **Federal Register** (77 FR 70584). A final rule implementing the Health Insurance Market Rules was published in the February 27, 2013 **Federal Register** (78 FR 13406) (2014 Market Rules).

A proposed rule relating to Exchanges and Insurance Market Standards for 2015 and Beyond was published in the March 21, 2014 **Federal Register** (79 FR 15808) (2015 Market Standards Proposed Rule). A final rule implementing the Exchange and Insurance Market Standards for 2015 and Beyond was published in the May 27, 2014 **Federal Register** (79 FR 30240) (2015 Market Standards Rule).

2. Exchanges

We published a request for comment relating to Exchanges in the August 3, 2010 **Federal Register** (75 FR 45584).

We issued initial guidance to States on Exchanges on November 18, 2010.[38] We issued a proposed rule in the July 15, 2011 **Federal Register** (76 FR 41865) to implement components of the Exchanges, and a proposed rule in the August 17, 2011 **Federal Register** (76 FR 51201) regarding Exchange functions in the individual market, eligibility determinations, and Exchange standards for employers. A final rule implementing components of the Exchanges and setting forth standards for eligibility for Exchanges was published in the March 27, 2012 **Federal Register** (77 FR 18309) (Exchange Establishment Rule).

In the March 8, 2016 **Federal Register** (81 FR 12203), we published the Patient Protection and Affordable Care Act; HHS Notice of Benefit and Payment Parameters for 2017 final rule (2017 Payment Notice), and established additional Exchange standards, including requirements for network adequacy and essential community providers; and established the timing of annual open enrollment periods.

In the September 6, 2016 **Federal Register** (81 FR 61456), we published the Patient Protection and Affordable Care Act; HHS Notice of Benefit and Payment Parameters for 2018 proposed rule (proposed 2018 Payment Notice). In the December 22, 2016 **Federal Register** (81 FR 94058), we published the Patient Protection and Affordable Care Act; HHS Notice of Benefit and Payment Parameters for 2018 final rule (2018 Payment Notice) and established additional Exchange standards, including requirements for network adequacy and essential community providers.

3. Special Enrollment Periods

In the July 15, 2011 **Federal Register** (76 FR 41865), we published a proposed rule establishing special enrollment periods for the Exchange. We implemented these special enrollment periods in the Exchange Establishment Rule (77 FR 18309). In the January 22, 2013 **Federal Register** (78 FR 4594), we published a proposed rule amending certain special enrollment periods, including the special enrollment periods described in §155.420(d)(3) and (7). We finalized these rules in the July 15, 2013 **Federal Register** (78 FR 42321).

In the June 19, 2013 **Federal Register** (78 FR 37032), we proposed to add a special enrollment period when the Exchange determines that a consumer has been incorrectly or inappropriately enrolled in coverage due to misconduct on the part of a non-Exchange entity. We finalized this proposal in the October 30, 2013 **Federal Register** (78 FR 65095). In the March 21, 2014 **Federal Register** (79 FR 15808), we proposed to amend various special enrollment periods. In particular, we proposed to clarify that later coverage effective dates for birth, adoption, placement for adoption, or placement for foster care would be effective the first of the month. The rule also proposed to clarify that earlier effective dates would be allowed if all issuers in an Exchange agree to effectuate coverage only on the first day of the specified month. Finally, this rule proposed adding that consumers may report a move in advance of the date of the move and established a special enrollment period for individuals losing medically needy coverage under the Medicaid program even if the medically needy coverage is not recognized as minimum essential coverage (individuals losing medically needy coverage that is recognized as minimum essential coverage already were eligible for a special enrollment period under the regulation). We finalized these provisions in the May 27, 2014 **Federal Register** (79 FR 30348). In the October 1, 2014 **Federal Register** (79 FR 59137), we published a correcting amendment related to codifying the coverage effective dates for plan selections made during a special enrollment period and clarifying a consumer's ability to select a plan 60 days before and after a loss of coverage.

In the November 26, 2014 **Federal Register** (79 FR 70673), we proposed to amend effective dates for special enrollment periods, the availability and length of special enrollment periods, the specific types of special enrollment periods, and the option for consumers to choose a coverage effective date of the first of the month following the birth, adoption, placement for adoption, or placement in foster care. We finalized these provisions in the February 27, 2015 **Federal Register** (80 FR 10866). In the July 7, 2015 **Federal Register** (80 FR 38653), we issued a correcting amendment to include those who become newly eligible for a QHP due to a release from incarceration. In the December 2, 2015 **Federal Register** (80 FR 75487) (proposed 2017 Payment Notice), we sought comment and data related to existing special enrollment periods, including data relating to the potential abuse of special enrollment periods. In the 2017 Payment Notice, we stated that in order to review the integrity of special enrollment periods, the Federally-facilitated Exchange (FFE) will conduct an assessment by collecting and reviewing documents from some consumers to confirm their eligibility for the special enrollment periods under which they enrolled.

In an interim final rule with comment published in the May 11, 2016 **Federal Register** (81 FR 29146), we amended the parameters of certain special enrollment periods.

In the 2018 Payment Notice, we established additional Exchange standards, including requirements for certain special enrollments.

4. Actuarial Value

On February 25, 2013, we established the requirements relating to EHBs and AVs in the Standards Related to Essential Health Benefits, Actuarial Value, and Accreditation Final Rule, which was published in the **Federal Register** (78 FR 12833) (EHB Rule), implementing section 1302 of the PPACA and 2707 of the PHS Act. In the 2018 Payment Notice published in the December 22, 2016 **Federal Register** (81 FR 94058), we finalized a provision that allows an expanded de minimis range for certain bronze plans.

B. Stakeholder Consultation and Input

HHS has consulted with stakeholders on policies related to the operation of Exchanges. We have held a number of listening sessions with consumers, providers, employers, health plans, the actuarial community, and State representatives to gather public input, with a particular focus on risks to the individual and small group markets, and how we can alleviate burdens facing patients and issuers. We consulted with stakeholders through regular meetings with the National Association of Insurance Commissioners, regular contact with States through the Exchange Establishment grant and Exchange Blueprint approval processes, and meetings with Tribal leaders and representatives, health insurance issuers, trade groups, consumer advocates, employers, and other interested parties.

III. Provisions of the Proposed

Regulations, and Analysis of and Responses to Public Comments

We published the "Patient Protection and Affordable Care Act; Market Stabilization" proposed rule in the February 17, 2017 **Federal Register** (82 FR 10980) (the proposed rule). We received 4,005 timely comments. The comments ranged from general support for or opposition to the proposed provisions to specific questions or comments regarding proposed changes. We received a number of comments and suggestions that were outside the scope of the proposed rule that will not be addressed in this final rule.

In this final rule, we provide a summary of each proposed provision, a summary of those public comments received that directly related to the proposals, our responses to them, and a description of the provisions we are finalizing.

Comment: We received comments stating that the comment period was unreasonably short, making it difficult for stakeholders to provide in-depth analysis and input. Some commenters stated that the short comment period represented a violation of the Administrative Procedure Act, 5 U.S.C. Ch. 5, Subch. II, sec. 551 *et seq.* Commenters suggested that HHS extend the comment period and provide a comment period of 30 or 60 days from the date of publication in the **Federal Register**.

Response: We published the proposed rule in order to promote issuer participation in the individual and small group markets and to address concerns raised by consumers, States, and issuers. While our general practice is to allow 30 to 60 days for comment, doing so is not specifically required by the Administrative Procedure Act. Because the changes directly affect issuers' plan designs and rates for 2018, HHS determined that it was necessary to have a 20-day comment period to finalize the rule in time for issuers to be able to factor the changes into their plans for the 2018 plan year. In addition, we believe that the short comment period was necessary to implement these changes in time to provide flexibility to issuers to help attract healthy consumers to enroll in health insurance coverage, improving the risk pool and bringing additional stability and certainty to the individual and small group markets for the 2018 plan year. Given the limited number of changes to existing rules contemplated by the proposed rule, we believe that the 20-day comment period provided adequate time for interested stakeholders to participate in the rulemaking process by submitting comments. The submission of more than 4,000 comments, many of which provided thoughtful, complex analyses of the proposals, suggests that the timeframe provided interested stakeholders with time to carefully consider and provide input on the proposals.

Comment: We received a number of comments in support of the proposed rule. Those commenters stated that the rule would stabilize and strengthen the risk pool by preventing gaming and encouraging full-year enrollment. In addition, those commenters stated that the proposals in the rule would benefit consumers by increasing coverage options, increasing consumer choice, and putting downward pressure on premiums, which would make coverage more affordable.

Response: We agree that the policies are expected to have a positive impact on stabilizing the markets, increasing consumer choice, and making coverage more affordable.

Comment: We received a number of comments discouraging HHS from finalizing the proposed rule. Some commenters stated that the rule was designed to benefit health insurance companies and would have an adverse impact on consumers' access to affordable health coverage. Commenters noted that they believed the rule would increase premiums and out-of-pocket costs, limit provider networks, and reduce covered benefits. Commenters also believed that the proposed rule would increase the number of uninsured and under-insured individuals. Furthermore, some commenters stated that the proposed rule would weaken the consumer protections offered under the PPACA, limit consumer choices, and limit patients' access to care. Those commenters also noted that the proposals would place undue administrative burdens on consumers and Exchanges. Many of these commenters suggested that additional changes to the Exchanges would cause further uncertainty and confusion for consumers and providers and encouraged HHS to wait to make any regulatory changes until Congress has passed new healthcare reform legislation.

Response: We appreciate the importance of ensuring that coverage purchased through the Exchanges is affordable to consumers, and believe affordability is critical to the success of the Exchanges. We understand commenters' concerns about loosening consumer protections, limiting patients' access to choices of coverage, and increasing administrative burdens. We note that this rule does not change the majority of standards for certification for QHPs, and agree that it is important to promote patients' access to quality coverage. Furthermore, we believe that this rule will improve the risk pools and help stabilize the individual and small group health insurance markets, which will help protect patients and consumers by encouraging issuers to maintain a presence in those markets and lower premiums, thereby increasing consumers' choices of affordable coverage options. We believe prompt regulatory action is necessary to stabilize the markets for the upcoming plan year, and recognize the importance of clearly communicating these changes in light of confusion and uncertainty for consumers and providers.

A. Part 147 – Health Insurance Reform Requirements for the Group and Individual Health Insurance Markets

1. Guaranteed Availability of Coverage (§147.104)

The guaranteed availability provisions at section 2702 of the PHS Act and §147.104 require health insurance issuers offering non-grandfathered coverage in the individual or group market to offer coverage to and accept every individual and employer in the State that applies for such coverage, unless an exception applies.[39] Individuals and employers typically are required to pay the first month's premium (sometimes referred to as a binder payment) before coverage is effectuated.

We have previously interpreted the guaranteed availability requirement to mean that an issuer is prohibited from applying a binder payment made for a new enrollment to past-due premiums[40] owed from any previous coverage and then refusing to effectuate the enrollment based on failure to pay premiums.[41] However, should the individual seek to renew existing coverage, the issuer could attribute the enrollee's forthcoming premium payments to any past-due premiums. In prior rulemaking related to the 2014 Market Rules, HHS received public comments expressing concerns about the potential for individuals with a history of non-payment to take unfair advantage of the guaranteed availability rules by declining to make premium payments, for example, at the end of a benefit year, yet being able to immediately sign up for new coverage for the next benefit year during the individual market open enrollment period.[42] In the preamble to the 2014 Market Rules, HHS encouraged States to consider approaches to discourage gaming and adverse selection while upholding consumers' guaranteed availability rights, and indicated an intention to address this issue in future guidance.

To address the concern about potential misuse of grace periods, we proposed to modify our interpretation of the guaranteed availability rules with respect to non-payment of premiums. Under the proposed rule, an issuer would not be considered to violate the guaranteed availability requirements if the issuer attributes a premium payment for coverage under the same or a different product to premiums due to the same issuer within the prior 12 months and refuses to effectuate new coverage for failure to pay premiums. To the extent permitted by applicable State law, this would permit an issuer to require an individual or employer to pay all past-due premiums owed to that issuer for coverage in the prior 12-month period in order to effectuate new coverage from that issuer. Under the proposed rule, an issuer choosing to adopt a policy of attributing payments in this way would be required to apply its premium payment policy uniformly to all employers or individuals in similar circumstances in the applicable market regardless of health status, and consistent with applicable non- discrimination requirements.[43] The proposal would not permit an issuer to condition the effectuation of new coverage on payment of premiums owed to a different issuer, or permit an issuer to condition the effectuation of new coverage on payment of past-due premiums by any individual other than the person contractually responsible for the payment of premium, as we do not believe it is reasonable to hold persons responsible for payments they were not contractually responsible for making. We stated that if the proposal were to be finalized, we would encourage States to adopt a similar approach, with respect to any State laws that might otherwise prohibit this practice.

Because of rules regarding grace periods and termination of coverage, individuals with past-due premiums would generally owe no more than 3 months of premiums.[8] Furthermore, for individuals on whose behalf the issuer received APTC, their past-due premiums would be net of any APTC that was paid on the individual's behalf to the issuer, with respect to any months for which the individual is paying past- due premiums.

We noted that due to operational constraints, the Federally-facilitated Small Business Health Options Program (FF–SHOP) would be unable to offer issuers this flexibility at this time. We solicited comments on the proposal, including on whether issuers that choose to adopt this type of premium payment policy should be permitted to implement it with a premium payment threshold policy, under which the issuer can consider an individual to have paid all amounts due, if the individual pays an amount, as determined by the issuer, that is less than the total past-due premiums. We also solicited comments on whether issuers should be required to provide notice to individuals regarding whether they have adopted a premium payment policy permitted under this proposal.

We are finalizing this proposal as follows. To the extent permitted by applicable State law, an issuer may attribute to any past-due premium amounts owed to that issuer the initial premium payment made in accordance with the terms of the health insurance policy to effectuate coverage. If the issuer is a member of a controlled group, the issuer may attribute any past- due premium amounts owed to any other issuer that is a member of such controlled group, for coverage in the 12- month period preceding the effective date of the new coverage when determining whether an individual or employer has made an initial premium payment to effectuate new coverage. Consistent with the scope of the guaranteed availability provision and subject to applicable State law, this policy applies both inside and outside of the Exchanges in the individual, small group, and large group markets,[44] and during applicable open enrollment or special enrollment periods. This policy does not permit a different issuer (other than one in the same controlled group as the issuer to which past-due premiums are owed) to condition the effectuation of new coverage on payment of past-due premiums or permit any issuer to condition the effectuation of new coverage on payment of past-due premiums by any individual other than the person contractually responsible for the payment of premiums.[45] As further described later in this preamble, for this purpose, the term controlled group means a group of two or more persons that is treated as a single employer under sections 52(a), 52(b), 414(m), or 414(o) of the Code. We also specify that issuers adopting this premium payment policy, as well as any issuers that do not adopt the policy but are within an adopting issuer's controlled group, must clearly describe in any enrollment application materials, and in any notice that is provided regarding non-payment of premiums, in paper or electronic form, the consequences of non-payment on future enrollment. We encourage States to adopt a similar approach; however, States may narrow the circumstances and conditions under which an issuer may apply a premium payment policy to past-due premiums before effectuating coverage or may prohibit the practice altogether.

[8]Section 156.270(d) requires issuers to observe a 3-consecutive month grace period before terminating coverage for those enrollees who upon failing to timely pay their premiums are receiving APTC. Section 155.430(d)(4) requires that when coverage is terminated following this grace period, the last day of enrollment in a QHP through the Exchange is the last day of the first month of the grace period. Therefore, individuals whose coverage is terminated at the conclusion of a grace period would owe at most 1 month of premiums, net of any APTC paid on their behalf

to the issuer. Individuals who attempt to enroll in new coverage while in a grace period (and whose coverage has not yet been terminated) could owe up to 3 months of premium, net of any APTC paid on their behalf to the issuer.

The following is a summary of the public comments we received on this proposal, and our responses.

Comment: Many commenters supported the proposal, suggesting that this approach is common in other industries such as housing, utilities, or telecommunications, where past-due payment for prior services must be made prior to restarting the same service. However, many other commenters objected to the proposal, stating that there is no statutory authority for the policy, that there is insufficient evidence of misuse of the grace period, and that individuals fail to make payments for a variety of other reasons, including poor or changing financial situations, poor health, or issuer or Exchange error. One commenter stated that the individual shared responsibility payment that is imposed for months in which non- exempt individuals do not have minimum essential coverage, as well as the fact that individuals have to pay for all of their healthcare expenses during any uninsured period, address any concerns about deliberate misuse of the grace period.

Other commenters who objected to the proposal stated that issuers have other ways, including collection actions, for recovering past-due premiums. Some of these commenters suggested that the individuals most likely to miss their premium payments are younger, healthier individuals, who could help balance the individual market risk pool. A few commenters stated that forcing individuals to pay retroactively for premiums covering months in which they did not seek healthcare will be a disincentive to signing up for coverage.

Response: We believe this interpretation of the guaranteed availability requirement will have a positive impact on the risk pool by removing economic incentives individuals may have had to pay premiums only when they were in need of healthcare services. We also believe this policy is an important means of encouraging individuals to maintain continuous coverage throughout the year and preventing abuses. While the guaranteed availability provision in section 2702 of the PHS Act does not explicitly refer to premium payment, it is clear from reading this provision together with the guaranteed renewability provision in section 2703 of the PHS Act that an issuer's sale and continuation in force of an insurance policy is contingent upon payment of premiums. We do not believe that the guaranteed availability provision is intended to require issuers to provide coverage to applicants who have not paid for such coverage. To the extent an individual or employer makes payment in the amount required to effectuate new coverage, but the issuer lawfully credits all or part of that amount toward past-due premiums, the consumer has not made sufficient initial payment for the new coverage.

With respect to individuals experiencing poor financial circumstances, we note that the PPACA provides for APTC and cost-sharing reductions (CSRs) for low-income individuals, and that increased APTC and CSRs are available as income decreases. We also note that consumers who experience a change in household income during a policy year are instructed to submit updated financial information to an Exchange and may potentially gain new, or additional, APTC or CSRs.

We disagree that the individual shared responsibility payment and paying for healthcare in the absence of coverage are sufficient to prevent abuses of the grace period, given that individuals may qualify for the short coverage gap exemption from the individual shared responsibility payment, and that individuals who misuse the grace period are likely to be individuals in good health who do not wish to make premium payments for periods of time during which they anticipate that they will not incur significant health expenses.

We acknowledge that issuers have ways of collecting debt other than by applying premium payments to past-due premiums. However, the policy in this regulation is intended to achieve a broader purpose than simply assisting issuers in collecting past-due premiums; rather this policy is intended to encourage individuals to maintain continuous coverage (and thereby avoid incurring past-due premiums) in order to help stabilize the risk pool for all participants, and prevent abuse of grace periods.

We believe the notice requirements discussed below, which will inform individuals of the consequences of missing their premium payments, will encourage younger, healthier individuals to maintain continuous coverage. Further, we disagree that requiring individuals to pay premiums owed for the months of prior coverage in which they did not seek healthcare will be a disincentive to signing up for coverage. We believe that with sufficient notice of having to pay past-due premiums before enrolling in new coverage, many individuals will instead opt to keep their coverage by making regular monthly premium payments.

Comment: Several commenters supported expanding the proposal. Some commenters stated that an issuer other than the specific licensed entity to which past-due premiums are owed, such as successors, assignees, commonly owned entities, other issuers within an Exchange, or any other issuer, should be permitted to refuse to effectuate new coverage as a result of unpaid past-due premiums. One commenter stated that limiting the proposal only to the specific licensed entity to which past-due premiums are owed will merely cause consumers to seek coverage from another issuer, thus limiting the policy's intended effect. Although several commenters agreed that the policy should not affect the ability of any individual other than the person contractually responsible for the payment of premiums to purchase coverage (such as the dependent of a policyholder, or an employee, when their employer has past-due premiums), several others commented that the policy should apply to the policyholder and to all covered dependents. For example, if a covered dependent of a former policyholder applies for new coverage, the issuer could refuse to effectuate new coverage for any individual in the enrollment group, unless past-due premiums are paid. Several commenters stated that the policy should permit issuers to collect all past-due premiums before effectuating coverage, even those for coverage beyond the past 12 months. Other commenters, however, suggested that a 12-month look-back is excessively punitive.

Response: In response to comments received, we believe that it will further the goals of this interpretation of guaranteed availability to allow the issuer to which past-due premiums are owed, and any other issuer that is a member of the same controlled group, to refuse to effectuate coverage unless the past-due premiums are paid. For this purpose, the term controlled group means a group of two or more persons that is treated as a single employer under sections 52(a), 52(b), 414(m), or 414(o) of the Code, which is the same definition used for other purposes related to the guaranteed renewability provision.[46] We believe this approach strikes a balance between comments suggesting a broad approach when premiums are owed to any issuer and comments favoring a narrow approach specific to premiums owed to the licensed entity. For now, we leave open the question of whether a successor or assignee issuer may take advantage of this flexibility to State interpretation, including in States where HHS is directly enforcing the guaranteed availability requirements. We believe that permitting an issuer to apply the policy to the dependent of a previous policyholder, when that dependent was covered under that previous policyholder's policy, or to an employee, when his or her employer was the previous policyholder, would be unreasonable, as it would require an individual or entity to pay a debt it has no legal obligation to pay. We also believe that a look-back period of 12 months (as opposed to a longer or shorter period) appropriately balances the objectives of the policy, without being unduly burdensome for consumers or carrying forward a debt owed for months beyond the previous year of coverage. We note that, although the look-back period is for 12 months, individuals with past-due premiums would generally owe no more than 1 to 3 months of premiums; they would not owe premiums for months in which they were not covered.

Comment: One commenter stated that Exchange assisters should inform consumers that if they wish to terminate their coverage, they should do so proactively, rather than simply fail to pay premiums.

Response: We encourage all entities and persons providing enrollment assistance, such as issuers, agents and brokers, Navigators, and other assisters, to educate consumers about how to terminate coverage so that it will not affect their ability to sign up for new coverage.

Comment: Many commenters stated that there should be a hardship exemption from the policy for individuals who are delinquent in their premiums for reasons other than gaming (such as domestic violence, falling victim to a crime, or issuer or Exchange error), and an appeals process for consumers to demonstrate hardship. A few commenters stated that any appeals process should include external review, or HHS review.

Response: States and issuers have the flexibility to create exemptions for extenuating circumstances, and appeals processes by which individuals and employers may demonstrate that they qualify for any such exemptions, as long as the policy is applied uniformly to individuals in similar circumstances in the applicable market within the State and not based on health status and consistent with applicable non- discrimination requirements. To the extent a State mandates an appeal or review process, it may also determine the logistics of that process.

Comment: Several commenters requested clarification that if an issuer collects past-due premiums, the issuer should be required to pay claims submitted for that individual during the grace period. They also stated that issuers should be required to immediately notify providers when an enrollee enters the grace period, so the providers could determine whether the providers would be penalized for furnishing non-urgent care, if past-due premiums are not paid. Another commenter stated that when past-due premiums are paid in full during a grace period, issuers should be required to pay all pended claims without the need for the provider to resubmit the claim or claims within 30 days of the enrollee's account becoming current. One commenter stated that if an issuer authorizes care and a provider provides care in reliance on that authorization, the issuer should be responsible for the claim, even if the claim would not otherwise be paid pursuant to the policy in this regulation.

Response: We clarify that issuers are required to pay all appropriate claims for services rendered to the enrollee during any months of coverage for which past-due premiums are collected. In the case of enrollees in the 3 consecutive month grace period, a QHP issuer must pay all appropriate claims for services rendered to the enrollee during the first month of the grace period, regardless of whether past-due premiums are paid, and must notify providers of the possibility for denied claims when an enrollee is in the second and third months of the grace period, as specified in §156.270(d). We are not modifying the rules regarding grace periods in this final rule. However, we will consider whether to make changes regarding provider notification requirements in the future.

Comment: We received several comments specific to loss of APTC. Several commenters stated that when individuals lose APTC for a period and then regain it, they have the right to choose whether they would like the APTC to be applied prospectively or retroactively. These commenters stated that Exchanges should be required to confirm with consumers if they would like the APTC to be applied retroactively, to reduce the amount of past-due premiums.

Response: Individuals generally must have their APTCs applied prospectively, and do not have a right to choose to have the APTC applied retroactively.

Only in limited circumstances, such as when an eligibility appeal determines that an Exchange erred in its determination of eligibility for APTC, are individuals permitted to have APTC applied retroactively. Where an individual's coverage through the Exchange has been terminated for non-payment of premiums, APTC is not available during any resulting coverage gap. While individuals may reapply for APTC to be applied prospectively,

APTC cannot be applied retroactively to periods during which the individual's coverage through the Exchange was terminated for non-payment of premiums. We note that individuals whose coverage is terminated at the conclusion of a grace period would owe premiums for the first month of the grace period, net of any APTC paid on their behalf to the issuer, but would not owe for the second and third months of the grace period, because the last day of enrollment in a QHP through the Exchange is the last day of the first month of the 3-month grace period, as outlined in §155.430(d)(4). Additionally, the individuals would not owe premiums for the months following termination.

Comment: Many commenters stated that issuers should be required to allow individuals to pay past-due premiums in installments, while the issuer sells them new coverage. One commenter stated that, during the installment period, consumers should be permitted to report any income changes, changes in household, or hardships, in order to make adjustments to the repayment plan.

Response: The policy in this final rule permits but does not require issuers to collect past-due premiums before effectuating new coverage. However, we are not requiring issuers that adopt the policy to accept installment payments in this final rule, although State law permitting or requiring issuers to accept such installment payments, as well as any requirements relating to notice of an adjustment to installment periods, would apply, provided the amount of installment payments an issuer will accept, and its decision whether or not to accept installment payments is applied uniformly to individuals or employers in similar circumstances in the applicable market within the State and not based on health status, and consistent with applicable non- discrimination requirements.

Comment: All commenters who commented on whether issuers should be permitted to accept a threshold amount of past-due premiums as payment in full supported this approach. One commenter stated that issuers that have a premium threshold for the binder and monthly premiums should not be required to do so for past- due premiums, and vice-versa. Another commenter stated that HHS should set a threshold that issuers should be required to accept. With respect to the disclosure of whether an issuer will accept a threshold, and the threshold amount, many commenters stated that issuers applying a payment threshold should be required to disclose the amount of the threshold either before purchase of the insurance policy, or at the time of enrollment. One commenter, however, stated that issuers should not be required to provide notice of a threshold, as such notice would incentivize partial payments.

Response: We decline to set a premium payment threshold or mandate that issuers set and apply one, or for those that do, require that they provide any such notice. Rather, issuers may set and apply a threshold to the extent permitted by applicable State law, provided that the issuer does so uniformly for individuals or employers in similar circumstances in the applicable market within the State and without regard to health status, and consistent with applicable non-discrimination requirements. Also, in accordance with the premium payment threshold regulation at §155.400(g) and guidance, issuers on an FFE, and on the State-based Exchanges on the Federal platform (SBE-FPs), that choose to apply a payment threshold policy must apply the policy in a uniform manner to all enrollees, and are expected to do so for the entire plan year.[47] Additionally under that regulation and guidance, if the issuer adopts such a policy, it is expected to apply the policy uniformly to the initial premium payment and any subsequent premium payments, and to any amount outstanding at the end of a grace period for non-payment of premium.

Comment: With respect to the comment solicitation regarding whether notice should be provided by issuers that adopt the premium payment policy, many commenters stated that such notice should be required. However, several commenters stated that no separate notice document is necessary. Rather, commenters stated that notice of the policy could be included on billing statements, any general payment policy notices, on the application, prior to purchase, or on issuers' Web sites. Commenters in favor of requiring notice stated that it should include the consequences of delinquent payment on the ability to purchase new coverage from the issuer, and other relevant information. Some commenters recommended this information appear in Plan Compare and in the Exchange eligibility determination notice.

Response: We agree that notice is important, but do not believe that a separate document is necessary, as issuers already have effective ways of communicating with consumers about premium payment. Therefore, we specify that issuers adopting a premium payment policy permitted under this section, as well as any other issuers that do not adopt the policy but are within an adopting issuer's controlled group, are required to clearly describe, in any enrollment application materials, and in any notice that is provided regarding non-payment of premiums, in paper or electronic form, the consequences of non-payment on future enrollment. We believe this notice is sufficient to inform consumers of their obligations to pay past-due premiums, and are not specifying additional notice in Plan Compare or in the Exchange eligibility determination at this time.

Comment: We received a few comments related to operationalizing the policy. One commenter stated that it would require information technology enhancements for an Exchange to process and store the industry standard code received from issuers that is sent when a consumer does not pay premiums. This would allow the issuer's system and enrollee's account to reflect the enrollment status with the issuer that elected to use their premium payment to satisfy past-due premiums. Due to the new interface requirements, the changes would be a large project and would consume a large amount of resources at considerable expense. Another commenter stated that the policy would require coordination between the Exchanges and issuers, and might require development in Exchanges' billing systems that would require time and resources for deployment. One commenter stated that the policy should be made optional because it is burdensome for issuers to reconcile 60 days of claims in order to reenroll individuals. One commenter asked for confirmation that the FFEs would operationalize the new policy by requiring issuers to send the Exchange a cancellation transaction for an enrollment of an individual who did not pay the outstanding balance by the applicable due date.

Response: As regards technical and operational challenges described by commenters related to permitting issuers to collect past-due premiums before effectuating new coverage, we note that nothing in this rule requires an issuer or Exchange to implement this type of premium payment policy before effectuating new coverage. We also note that these challenges are only applicable to Exchanges that perform premium collection on behalf of issuers, such as the FF-SHOP, which due to operational limitations, is not able to implement the policy at this time. As regards comments about processing enrollment- related transactions, we note that QHP issuers are currently required to communicate to the FFE and to SBE- FPs whether an enrollment is effectuated or cancelled, such as when the individual fails to make sufficient payment to effectuate new coverage.

Comment: One commenter stated that the policy should apply only to individuals who enter the grace period, and to past-due premiums accrued, after the effective date of the final rule.

Response: For issuers that choose to adopt the premium payment policy, and for other issuers in such an issuer's controlled group, the requirement to provide notice of the policy will become effective beginning with notices provided 60 days after publication of the final rule. Beginning on or after that date, issuers will not be considered to violate Federal guaranteed availability requirements if they attribute payments toward past-due premiums consistent with this section and then deny enrollment for failure to pay the initial payment for a new enrollment to individuals to whom such notice was provided prior to their failure to pay premiums that become past-due premiums.

In addition to the policy on past-due premiums, we proposed to amend §147.104(b)(2)(i) to conform to proposed changes to special enrollment periods discussed in greater detail in section III.B.2. of the proposed rule (82 FR 10984). Because the proposed changes to §155.420(a)(4) and (5) applied to special enrollment periods in the individual market, both inside and outside of an Exchange, we proposed to amend §147.104(b)(2)(i) to specify that these paragraphs apply to special enrollment periods throughout the individual market. We solicited comments on how these changes would be operationalized outside of theExchanges.

B. *Part 155 – Exchange Establishment Standards and Other Related Standards Under the Patient Protection and Affordable Care Act*

1. Enrollment of Qualified Individuals Into QHPs (§155.400)

We are finalizing an amendment to §155.400 to address binder payment requirements that apply when a consumer whose enrollment was delayed due to an eligibility verification opts to delay the coverage start date under §155.420(b)(5). A more detailed discussion of the pre-enrollment verification procedures for special enrollment periods and the related changes that we are finalizing in §155.400 are provided in section III.B.3 of this final rule.

2. Initial and Annual Open Enrollment Periods (§155.410)

We proposed to amend paragraph (e) of §155.410, which provides the dates for the annual Exchange open enrollment period in which qualified individuals and enrollees may apply for or change coverage in a QHP. The Exchange open enrollment period is extended by cross-reference to non-grandfathered plans in the individual market, both inside and outside of an Exchange, under guaranteed availability regulations at §147.104(b)(1)(ii). In prior rulemaking, we established that the open enrollment period for the benefit year beginning on January 1, 2018, would begin on November 1, 2017 and extend through January 31, 2018; and that the open enrollment period for the benefit years beginning on January 1, 2019 and beyond would begin on November 1 and extend through December 15 of the calendar year preceding the benefit year.[14] We noted at the time that we believe that, as the Exchanges continue, a month-and-a-half open enrollment period provides sufficient time for consumers to enroll in or change QHPs for the upcoming benefit year. Furthermore, this timeframe would achieve our goals of shifting to an earlier open enrollment end date, so that all consumers who enroll during this time will receive a full year of coverage, which will increase access for patients and simplify operational processes for issuers and the Exchanges. In addition, we noted that we also believe that this shorter open enrollment period may have a positive impact on the risk pool because it will reduce opportunities for adverse selection by those who learn that they will need healthcare services in late December or January. Although we originally thought a longer transition period was needed before moving to this shorter open enrollment period, in the proposed rule, we stated that we believe that the market and issuers are now ready for this adjustment sooner. Therefore, we proposed to amend §155.410(e) to change the open enrollment period for benefit year 2018 so that it begins on November 1, 2017 and runs through December 15, 2017. All consumers who select plans on or before December 15, 2017 would receive an enrollment effective date of January 1, 2018, as already required by §155.410(f)(2)(i). We noted that we believe that this open enrollment period would align better with many open enrollment periods for employer-based coverage, as well as the open enrollment period for Medicare Advantage.

We solicited comments on this proposal, in particular on the capacity of State Exchanges (SBEs) to shift to the shorter open enrollment period for the 2018 benefit year, on the effect of the shorter enrollment period on issuers' ability to enroll healthy consumers, and any difficulties agents, brokers, Navigators, and other assisters may have in serving consumers seeking to enroll during this shorter time period.

We are finalizing this provision as proposed.

Comment: Many commenters supported our proposal to shift the open enrollment period end date to December 15, 2017 for the 2018 benefit year. These commenters noted that this change will improve the risk pool by encouraging people to maintain coverage and preventing adverse selection from partial-year enrollments, as well as eliminate operational complexity for issuers. Several of these commenters stated that a uniform January 1 coverage start date is an important element in promoting continuous, full-year coverage, and will help prevent gaming by healthy individuals who wait until the end of open enrollment to enroll in coverage with a later effective date, which would help issuers manage risk and develop appropriate rates with consumers enrolled for the full year.

A large number of commenters expressed concerns with our proposal. Among these commenters, many worried that a shorter open enrollment period would reduce enrollment overall. These commenters disagreed that a shorter open enrollment period would reduce premiums or improve the health of the risk pool. Instead, they were concerned that it would discourage enrollment by young and healthy consumers, who typically wait until the end of open enrollment to enroll. Others disagreed with the proposal that it was important that the open enrollment timeframe mirror employer-sponsored insurance, pointing out that the enrollees in employer-sponsored insurance have different characteristics from Exchange enrollees and the process for enrolling in health coverage is markedly different.

Response: After consideration of the comments received, we are finalizing an open enrollment period for the 2018 benefit year that begins on November 1, 2017 and runs through December 15, 2017. We had already planned to implement a consistent month-and-a- half open enrollment period beginning with open enrollment for the 2019 benefit year; therefore, we believe that implementing the same open enrollment timeframe 1 year earlier will not increase the burden on consumers or make it harder to enroll. As we have previously stated, shifting to an earlier open enrollment period closing date ensures that consumers who enroll during this time will receive a full year of coverage, which will reduce adverse selection risk for issuers.[48] We agree with commenters who noted that ending the open enrollment period on December 15, 2017, for the 2018 benefit year will decrease operational complexity and cost for issuers, since the coverage start date for all enrollments (other than those pursuant to a special enrollment period) will be on the same day (January 1, 2018), and the Exchange open enrollment period will align better with that for employer-based and Medicare Advantage plans. We intend to conduct outreach to consumers to ensure that they are aware that the deadline for enrolling in coverage during the open enrollment period has changed and recognize the importance of targeting young and healthy individuals who, as commenters noted, often wait until close to the deadline to enroll.

Comment: Commenters both in favor of and opposed to the proposed timeframe expressed concern about the burden a shortened open enrollment period could create on the Exchanges and on other resources. These commenters warned that because a greater number of people will be trying to enroll at the same time, Exchanges must increase technology infrastructure and capacity to accommodate this shorter open enrollment period. Commenters stated that implementing this shorter timeframe a year earlier than previously planned does not allow Exchanges sufficient time to work out glitches and fix errors. Some commenters were concerned that agents, brokers, Navigators, and other assisters would be overwhelmed with such a short period of time to assist consumers. Among these commenters, some recommended enhanced funding for Navigators and other assisters, so that they could produce the same quality of assistance in a shorter timeframe. Some commenters worried that the overlap of the Exchange open enrollment period with the Medicare Advantage open enrollment period may confuse consumers, or strain the capacity of agents and brokers. Other commenters expressed concern that a compressed open enrollment period would increase the administrative and marketing burden on issuers, resulting in an increase in administrative costs. Several commenters were concerned that State budgets could not accommodate additional outreach or technology expenditures for the next open enrollment period.

Many commenters worried that the proposed timeframe would cause confusion and hardship for consumers, particularly during the winter holidays and towards the end of school semesters. Some commenters worried that consumers would not have sufficient time to respond to outreach and advertising, review and compare plans and make informed decisions about their coverage, or have their documentation ready and their information verified by an Exchange. Many commenters stated that younger populations, consumers with limited English proficiency, low-income communities, rural communities, and first-time enrollees need more time to process and understand coverage options. Many commenters sought greater specificity on HHS's outreach plans, and encouraged additional education and marketing efforts to ensure that consumers are aware of the shortened open enrollment period.

Response: We believe that shifting the open enrollment period end date to December 15, 2017, for the 2018 benefit year provides sufficient time for all entities involved in the annual open enrollment process to conduct outreach, provide assistance, or enroll in coverage. We intend to conduct outreach to consumers to ensure that they are aware of the newly shortened open enrollment period in advance of the November 1, 2017, start date and are prepared to enroll or re-enroll in 2018 coverage.

We agree with commenters that, because of the compressed timeframe, consumers may require additional assistance with submitting requested documents and choosing the plan that works best for them. We note that many Navigators already focus on the populations who may require this additional help, such as consumers with limited English proficiency and low-income and rural communities. *Comment:* Many commenters recommended providing State flexibility to determine open enrollment period timeframes. Other commenters recommended alternative open enrollment period timeframes. Among these commenters, some recommended maintaining the current open enrollment period from November 1 through January 31. Other commenters proposed alternative open enrollment periods lasting from November 1 through December 31, from October 1 through December 15, from January 1 through February 15, or from November 1 to April 15 to align with the tax season. Some commenters recommended structuring open enrollment periods around consumers' birth month, similar to traditional Medicare enrollment, or by consumers' last name. Lastly, other commenters recommended that we allow enrollment year-round.

Response: We believe that a consistent, nationwide, individual market open enrollment period will help prevent consumer confusion and reduce administrative complexity for issuers, agents, brokers, Navigators and other assisters who serve States with FFEs and States with SBEs. Shifting the start date of open enrollment prior to November 1 for the 2018 benefit year would not allow Exchanges, issuers, or assisters adequate time to prepare for open enrollment. Instead, we believe implementing the same open enrollment timeframe for the 2018 benefit year as we will implement for the 2019 benefit year and beyond will help promote stability in the Exchanges and consistency across benefit years. However, we recognize that some SBEs may have operational difficulties this year in transitioning to this shorter open enrollment period. Under their existing regulatory authority, those Exchanges may elect to supplement the open enrollment period with a special enrollment period, as a transitional measure, to account for those operational difficulties.

We intend to closely monitor the implementation of this open enrollment period and will consider whether we should shift to an earlier open enrollment period start date of either October 1 or October 15 for future open enrollment periods.

3. Special Enrollment Periods (§155.420)

Section 1311(c)(6) of the PPACA establishes enrollment periods, including special enrollment periods, for qualified individuals for enrollment in QHPs through an Exchange. Section 1311(c)(6)(C) of the PPACA states that the Secretary is to provide for special enrollment periods specified in section 9801 of the Code and other special enrollment periods under circumstances similar to such periods under part D of title XVIII of the Act. Section 2702(b)(3) of the PHS Act also directs the Secretary to provide for market-wide special enrollment periods for qualifying events under section 603 of the Employee Retirement Income Security Act of 1974.

Special enrollment periods are a longstanding feature of employer-sponsored coverage. They exist to ensure that people who lose health coverage during the year (for example, through non-voluntary loss of minimum essential coverage provided through an employer), or who experience other qualifying events, such as marriage or the birth or adoption of a child, have the opportunity to enroll in new coverage or make changes to their existing coverage. In the individual market, while the annual open enrollment period allows previously uninsured individuals to enroll in new coverage, special enrollment periods are intended, in part, to promote continuous enrollment in health coverage during the benefit year by allowing those who were previously enrolled in coverage to obtain new coverage without a lapse or gap in coverage.

Our past practice, in many cases, was to permit individuals seeking coverage through the Exchanges to self-attest to their eligibility for most special enrollment periods and to enroll in coverage without further verification of their eligibility or without submitting proof of prior coverage. This practice had the virtue of minimizing barriers to obtaining coverage for consumers, which can, in particular, deter enrollment by healthy individuals. However, as the Government Accountability Office noted in a November 2016 report, relying on self- attestation without verifying documents submitted to show a special enrollment period triggering event could allow applicants to obtain subsidized coverage for which they would otherwise not qualify.[49] In addition, allowing previously uninsured individuals who elected not to enroll in coverage during the annual open enrollment period to instead enroll in coverage through a special enrollment period for which they would not otherwise qualify during the benefit year, undermines the incentive for enrolling in a full year of coverage through the annual open enrollment period and increases the risk of adverse selection from individuals who wait to enroll until they are sick. Such behaviors can create a sicker risk pool, leading to higher rates and reduced availability of coverage.

a. Pre-Enrollment Verification of Special Enrollment Period Eligibility

In an effort to curb abuses of special enrollment periods, in 2016 we added warnings on HealthCare.gov regarding inappropriate use of special enrollment periods. We also eliminated several special enrollment periods and tightened certain eligibility rules.[50] Also in 2016, we announced retrospective audits of a random sampling of enrollments through loss of minimum essential coverage and permanent move special enrollment periods, 2 commonly used special enrollment periods. Additionally, we created a special enrollment confirmation process under which consumers enrolling through common special enrollment periods were directed to provide documentation to confirm their eligibility.[51] Finally, we proposed to implement (beginning in June 2017) a pilot program for conducting pre-enrollment verification of eligibility for certain special enrollment periods.[52]

As discussed in the 2018 Payment Notice, the impact of special enrollment period verification on risk pools may be complex. Some commenters suggested that additional steps to determine special enrollment period eligibility worsen the problem by creating new barriers to enrollment, with healthier, less motivated individuals, the most likely to be deterred. The pilot was initially planned to sample 50 percent of consumers who were attempting to newly enroll in Exchange coverage through certain special enrollment periods in order to provide a statistically sound method to compare the claims experience in the second half of 2017 between individuals subject to pre-enrollment verification with those who were not.

However, based on strong issuer feedback and the potential to help stabilize the market for 2018 coverage, we proposed to increase the scope of pre-enrollment verification of special enrollment periods to all applicable special enrollment periods in order to ensure complete verification of eligibility. We proposed to begin to implement this expanded pre- enrollment verification starting in June 2017. We have consistently heard from issuers and other stakeholders that pre-enrollment verification of special enrollment periods is critical to promote continuous coverage, protect the risk pool, and stabilize rates. We agree that policies and practices that allow individuals to remain uninsured and wait to enroll in coverage through a special enrollment period only after becoming sick can contribute to market destabilization and reduced issuer participation, which can reduce the availability of coverage for individuals.

Therefore, we proposed that HHS conduct pre-enrollment verification of eligibility for Exchange coverage for applicable categories of special enrollment periods for all new consumers in all States served by the HealthCare.gov platform, which includes FFEs and SBE-FPs.

Under pre-enrollment verification, HHS would verify eligibility for new consumers who seek to enroll in Exchange coverage through applicable special enrollment periods. Consumers would be able to submit their applications and select a QHP; then, as is the current practice for most special enrollment periods, the start date of that coverage would be determined by the date of QHP selection. However, the consumers' enrollment would be "pended" until the Exchange completes verification of their special enrollment period eligibility. In this context, "pending" means the Exchange will hold the information regarding QHP selection and coverage start date until special enrollment period eligibility is confirmed, and only then release the enrollment information to the relevant issuer. Consumers would have 30 days from the date of QHP selection to provide documentation, and could either upload documents into their account on HealthCare.gov or send their documents in the mail.

When possible, we intend to make every effort to verify an individual's eligibility for the applicable special enrollment period through automated electronic means instead of through consumer-submitted documentation. For example, we would verify a birth by confirming the baby's existence through existing electronic verifications or electronically verify that a consumer was denied Medicaid or CHIP coverage, where such information is available. Otherwise, we intend to seek documentation from the individual applying for coverage through the special enrollment period. We noted that, even though we do not currently perform verification for all consumers new to the Exchange, we already require all consumers to provide documentation if they are applying for coverage through a special enrollment period based on certain qualifying events. As proposed, we anticipate approximately the same amount of documentation under the rule that is currently required, and therefore, would not anticipate an increased burden on consumers. We solicited comments on the impact on consumers. We also solicited comments on our proposed method for pre- enrollment verification and whether we should retain a small percentage of enrollees outside of the pre-enrollment verification process to conduct the study discussed above. We noted that if we do not, HHS would continue to monitor other indicators of risk where available, in lieu of the statistical comparison. Recognizing that pre- enrollment verification could have the unintended consequence of deterring healthier individuals from purchasing Exchange coverage, we also solicited comments on what strategies HHS should take to increase the chances that these individuals complete the verification process.

In addition, we recommended that SBEs that do not currently conduct pre- enrollment verification of special enrollment period eligibility consider following this approach as well, and requested comment on whether SBEs should also be required to conduct pre-enrollment verification, with an appropriate amount of time to implement such a process, and how long that transition period should be. We are moving forward with a pre- enrollment verification of eligibility for applicable special enrollment periods as proposed. This initiative will include all States served by the HealthCare.gov platform, which includes FFEs and SBE-FPs. We note that implementation of pre-enrollment verification of special enrollment periods in these States will be phased in, focusing first on the categories with the highest volume and of most concern—such as loss of minimum essential coverage, permanent move, Medicaid/CHIP denial, marriage, and adoption. We intend to closely monitor the effectiveness of pre- enrollment verification methods for those categories of special enrollment periods and will continue to adjust and improve our verification processes in order to ensure accurate determinations of eligibility for all special enrollment periods.

SBEs maintain flexibility to determine whether and how to implement a pre- enrollment verification of eligibility for special enrollment periods. For example, an SBE could consider allowing issuers to conduct the verification, if the SBE itself is unable to implement pre-enrollment verification.

Comment: Commenters expressed concern about the proposal to conduct pre-enrollment verification of eligibility for special enrollment periods, which they fear will increase barriers to enrollment and deter consumers, especially young and healthy consumers, from enrolling in coverage, which will worsen the risk pool. Commenters stated that consumers with ongoing medical needs will spend the time and effort needed to submit documentation, but those without a current or ongoing need for healthcare services or who do not have documents readily available or easily accessible, will be more likely to forgo verifying their eligibility for a special enrollment period. Citing a study that estimated that only 5 percent of eligible consumers enroll through special enrollment periods during the year,[53] commenters expressed concern that special enrollment periods are already underutilized and expressed fear that instituting a pre-enrollment verification of eligibility will further reduce the percentage of eligible consumers enrolling through special enrollment periods. Commenters cited early results from a 2016 HHS study of post- enrollment verification of special enrollment periods, which reported a 20 percent decrease in special enrollment period enrollments compared to the same time period in 2015, and found that applications with younger household contacts were less likely to verify their special enrollment periods.[54] These commenters warned that pre-enrollment verification of special enrollment period eligibility could have a greater impact across both of these measures.

In addition to consumers opting not to submit documents, commenters noted that other groups of consumers, such as those in rural areas, low-income workers, immigrants, and those with limited English proficiency, will likely be disproportionately impacted by a pre-enrollment verification and may experience difficulty submitting their documents, even if qualifying for a special enrollment period and being motivated to enroll in and start new health coverage. These commenters noted that external variables, such as the distance to the nearest assister, agent, or broker; difficulty taking time off work; difficulty obtaining needed documents; or confusion about which documents to submit and how, all affect consumers' ability to submit documents. For example, commenters maintained that farm workers often have difficulty documenting that they moved and consumers living in rural areas may be unable to easily copy or upload documents. For the special enrollment periods for loss of minimum essential coverage and permanent move, commenters raised concerns that even though consumers may be enrolled or recently enrolled in coverage, they may still have difficulty submitting documents due to the fact that issuers and health plans are no longer required to send enrollees certificates of credible coverage (commenters requested that this prior HIPAA requirement be reinstated) and due to printing and re- printing delays at State Medicaid agencies. Other commenters mentioned that the event that qualifies the consumer for a special enrollment period, such as a permanent move, may itself impair the consumer's ability to submit required documentation on time. Therefore, several commenters requested that the document submission deadline be extended from 30 to 60 or 90 days, and that consumers be able to request a deadline extension if they are having difficulty gathering documents.

In addition to concerns about consumers' ability to gather and submit needed documents, commenters expressed concerns about possible delays in enrollment due to system issues, processing backlogs, and long wait times, confusion, or lack of information at the Exchange call center. Commenters were concerned that these delays could have serious negative health consequences for consumers, especially children. Several commenters requested that the FFE exclude from pre-enrollment verification any special enrollment periods that are often used to enroll children, such as the special enrollment periods for birth, adoption, foster care placement, court order, and Medicaid or CHIP denial.

Commenters noted that there are still many unknowns about the consumers who enroll in coverage through special enrollment periods, including a lack of evidence demonstrating misuse and abuse. In addition, commenters observed, that to the extent that misuse and abuse exist, it is unclear whether requiring pre-enrollment verification will serve as an effective deterrent. Some commenters requested that we share this data before proceeding with pre-enrollment verification or that we continue to collect data about consumer behavior by continuing with post- enrollment verification of eligibility for special enrollment periods. Other commenters stated that, if the FFE is to proceed with pre-enrollment verification of eligibility for special enrollment periods, it should proceed with caution by rolling it out slowly, in order to permit sufficient education of stakeholders and other entities involved, to address any unanticipated technical or other issues that may arise, and to collect robust data about impacted consumers. Many of these commenters recommended that the FFE start with a randomly selected pilot that would subject 50 percent of applicants attempting to enroll through a special enrollment period to pre-enrollment verification, as originally planned, while other commenters recommended proceeding with a 90 percent pilot, assuming the remaining 10 percent constitute a statistically significant control group.

In contrast, other commenters support conducting a pre-enrollment verification of eligibility for all applicants attempting to enroll through a special enrollment period. These commenters noted that pre-enrollment verification is the existing standard in the small group market, so it makes sense to apply the same standard to the individual market. Commenters requested that HHS establish consistent standards for verifying eligibility both across special enrollment periods and across markets, so that consumers are treated the same. Several issuers requested that the FFE agree to share collected documents with issuers at their request in order to assist with verifying enrollments outside of the Exchange. These commenters stated that performing pre-enrollment verification of eligibility for all special enrollment periods is a necessary next step to deter bad actors and prevent misuse and abuse of special enrollment periods. Doing so, commenters stated, will drive down premium costs in the future, which will benefit consumers across the individual market.

Commenters who supported robust pre-enrollment verification of eligibility for special enrollment periods stated that it was not necessary to exclude any consumers from being subject to pre- enrollment verification and urged us to proceed with verifying 100 percent of consumers attempting to enroll in coverage through a special enrollment period. Some commenters stated that we could use enrollment data from the past 2 years as a control group for the purpose of measuring any potential consumer impact of a pre-enrollment verification of eligibility.

Response: We appreciate commenters' concerns about the potential impact that pre-enrollment verification may have on young and healthy consumers, and their decision about whether to complete the steps needed to verify their eligibility. We are acutely aware of the importance of attracting healthy consumers to the individual market, and Exchanges in particular, in order to stabilize and improve the risk pool. As we implement pre-enrollment verification, we will seek to monitor enrollments by different groups of individuals affected by this process to determine its impact. In addition, we appreciate the concerns that certain consumers, especially vulnerable populations, may face barriers to gathering and timely submitting documents, and that delays in enrollment can have a negative impact on consumers', especially children's, health. We plan to conduct trainings for both internal and external stakeholders, so that they understand what the new pre-enrollment verification requirements are, what information will be available, and how to successfully prove one's eligibility for each special enrollment period where documentation will be required. We are also committed to expediting review of these documents to minimize any delay, and will be equipping our call center with frequent status updates in order to assist in answering questions that may arise.

We understand that consumers may not currently possess or may require time to gather the necessary documents to verify their eligibility, and intend to exercise reasonable flexibility with respect to the documentation required under this policy. We believe that documentation is likely to be most difficult for consumers who qualify for the loss of minimum essential coverage, permanent move, or Medicaid or CHIP denial special enrollment periods. Therefore, we will permit consumers to send us the details about their qualifying event with an explanation of why they are unable to submit requested documentation, and we will take their letters into consideration when deciding whether to exercise reasonable flexibility. In addition, in response to the comments regarding certificates of credible coverage, we note that under sections 1502 and 1514 of the PPACA and section 6055 of the Code, enrollees have proof of previous year health coverage via their tax statements, which may be helpful in some circumstances. We also note that the Exchanges will accept many other types of documentation from consumers seeking to verify their prior coverage, including letters from insurers, employers, and government health programs.

Despite the concerns raised, we believe that in order to help stabilize the individual market, we must implement a robust pre-enrollment verification of eligibility for special enrollment periods where new consumers will have their eligibility verified. This will help ensure that consumers are not misusing special enrollment periods, which we anticipate will both improve the risk pool and reduce premiums for all Exchange enrollees. Therefore, we are proceeding as proposed to implement pre- enrollment verification of eligibility for special enrollment periods beginning in June 2017. Stakeholders will receive additional updates from us in the coming months.

Comment: Commenters supported using electronic verification, to the extent possible, to verify eligibility for special enrollment periods. Commenters stated that using electronic data sources will minimize any potential burden on consumers seeking to enroll and any delays in starting their coverage. A few commenters requested that the FFE wait to begin a pre-enrollment verification of eligibility until methods for electronically verifying eligibility for all special enrollment periods were in place. Other commenters requested that we continue to explore the use of additional electronic data sources, and several issuers offered to work with us on this effort. Absent a streamlined method for electronic verification of all special enrollment periods, commenters expressed concerns about the lack of Federal staff and resources available to adjudicate documents in a timely manner, especially when the work is layered on top of ongoing post-enrollment documentation verification for inconsistencies. Commenters noted the increased costs to the Federal government due to increased staffing needs and secure storage of submitted documents, and the additional time both consumers and assisters will need to spend to adhere to these new requirements. A few commenters indicated that a pre-enrollment verification of special enrollment period eligibility may also affect other entities, such as issuers and medical providers who would incur costs in re-submitting or refiling claims, processing retroactive claims, and effectuating retroactive enrollments. One commenter suggested that HHS's cost analysis include these costs, as well as the consumer cost of spending time requesting that claims be re-billed.

Response: We appreciate commenters' support for using electronic data sources, to the extent possible, to verify eligibility for special enrollment periods, and agree that the use of electronic data sources will minimize the burden on consumers and facilitate faster verifications. For these reasons, we intend to make every effort to verify an individual's eligibility for the applicable special enrollment period through automated electronic means when possible. Furthermore, we are exploring ways to enhance and expand our use of electronic verification to other special enrollment periods in the near future. We hope to minimize any burden on other stakeholders by swiftly reviewing any verification documents received and releasing pended enrollments as quickly as possible.

We appreciate the concerns about the increased burden and cost that a documentation requirement for pre- enrollment verification of eligibility for special enrollment periods will have on all entities involved. We are dedicated to reviewing all special enrollment period documents received as quickly as possible in order to minimize delays. Although we recognize that gathering and submitting these documents can be difficult and time consuming, we do not believe that this places a new burden on consumers and those providing enrollment assistance since consumers are already required to submit documentation to prove their eligibility after enrollment for 5 common special enrollment periods. Because of our plans for timely document review, we do not believe that new costs will be incurred by issuers, medical providers, or consumers needing to re-submit, refile, or re-bill for claims for services received due to this new requirement.

Comment: Many commenters requested that States be provided flexibility on whether and how to implement a pre-enrollment verification of eligibility for special enrollment periods. Several States commented that they already have procedures and policies in place to verify eligibility for special enrollment periods, and would prefer to continue using methods that make sense for their State. Commenters also expressed concern about the technical build that would be required for SBEs to mirror the proposed process for FFEs and SBE-FPs, and several States commented that they do not think they could be ready for a June 2017 implementation date. Commenters who supported requiring SBEs to conduct a pre-enrollment verification of eligibility for enrollment through special enrollment periods expressed an interest in standardizing requirements and processes across Exchanges, so that all consumers are held to the same standards and treated the same.

Response: While we appreciate the benefits of consistency across Exchanges and markets to ensure fair and equal treatment of consumers, we believe it is important to provide States with flexibility to adopt policies that fit the needs of their State, and will not require a State to conduct pre-enrollment verification. However, we encourage SBEs to implement pre-enrollment verification as soon as possible, and hope that they will utilize creative and innovative methods to do so, including allowing issuers to perform the verification on behalf of the SBE. In addition, we recognize that several SBEs have already made progress in developing methods for verifying eligibility for special enrollment periods.

b. Special Enrollment Period Limitations for Existing Enrollees

As noted above, the pre-enrollment verification of special enrollment period eligibility is intended to address concerns about potential adverse selection among qualified individuals who are new to the Exchanges. However, we have heard concerns that existing Exchange enrollees are utilizing special enrollment periods to change plan metal levels based on health needs that emerge during the benefit year, and that this is having a negative impact on the risk pool. As discussed in the proposed rule, we have concerns about pending a new enrollment until pre- enrollment verification is conducted for current Exchange enrollees, who would still have an active policy. We believe the potential overlap of current, active policies and pended new enrollments would cause significant confusion for consumers and create burdens on issuers with respect to managing the potential operational issues. For example, if a current enrollee seeks to add a new spouse under the marriage special enrollment period, the current coverage would generally remain in force until the consumer submits documentation to verify the marriage. At that time, the pended new enrollment for both individuals would be released, potentially with a retroactive coverage effective date based on the date of the plan selection, and the current coverage with the single enrollee would be retroactively terminated to when the new policy begins. If the new plan selection is with a new issuer, any claims incurred during the time period the new enrollment is pended would need to be reconciled across the issuers.

As an alternative to performing pre- enrollment verification of special enrollment period eligibility for existing Exchange enrollees, we proposed to limit the ability of existing Exchange enrollees to change plan metal levels during the benefit year. This proposed change was reflected in regulatory text by proposed revisions to the introductory text of

§155.420(d), and the proposed additions of paragraphs (a)(3) and (4) to §155.420. We proposed that paragraph (a)(4) would also apply in the individual market outside the Exchanges, but would not apply in the group market. We proposed changes to §§147.104(b)(2)(i) and 155.725(j)(2)(i) to specify this. We solicited comments on all aspects of the proposal, including whether it would be preferable to address adverse selection concerns for existing enrollees by applying the approach of pending plan selections until pre-enrollment verification is completed based on document reviews instead of the proposed restrictions based on current plan and metal level. We also solicited comments on any alternative strategies for addressing potential adverse selection issues for existing enrollees who are eligible for a special enrollment period.

We understand that SBEs may not be able to implement these changes starting in 2017, and sought comments on an appropriate transitional period for SBEs, or whether these changes should be optional for SBEs.

Under new paragraph (a)(4)(i) of §155.420, we proposed to require that, if an enrollee qualifies for a special enrollment period due to gaining a dependent as described in paragraph (d)(2)(i), the Exchange may allow him or her to add the new dependent to his or her current QHP (subject to the ability to enroll in silver level coverage in certain circumstances as discussed in the next paragraph). Alternatively, if the QHP's business rules do not allow the new dependent to enroll (for example, because the QHP is only available as self-only coverage), the Exchange may allow the enrollee and his or her new dependent to enroll in another QHP within the same level of coverage (or an "adjacent" level of coverage, if no such plans are available), as defined in §156.140(b). Alternatively, new dependents may enroll by themselves in a separate QHP at any metal level. This proposal sought to ensure that enrollees who qualify for the special enrollment period due to gaining a dependent are using this special enrollment period for its primary purpose of enrolling the new dependent in coverage. We stated in the proposed rule that, if finalized, we intended to implement this policy for the FFEs and SBE–FPs as soon as practicable.

Section 155.420(a)(4)(ii) proposed to require that if an enrollee or his or her dependent is not enrolled in a silver level QHP and becomes newly eligible for cost-sharing reductions and qualifies for the special enrollment periods in paragraphs (d)(6)(i) and (ii) of §155.420, the

Exchange may allow the enrollee and dependent to enroll in a QHP at the silver level, as specified in §156.140(b)(2), if they choose to change their QHP enrollment. We solicited comments on this proposal, including with respect to whether individuals newly eligible for APTC who qualify for the special enrollment periods at §155.420(d)(6)(i) and (ii) should also be able to enroll in a silver level QHP, or QHPs at other metal levels.

Paragraph (a)(4)(iii) of §155.420 proposed that, for an enrollee who qualifies for the remaining special enrollment periods specified in paragraph (d), the Exchange generally need only allow the enrollee and his or her dependents to make changes to their enrollment in the same QHP or to change to another QHP within the same level of coverage, as defined in §156.140(b), if other QHPs at that metal level are available. This restriction would extend to enrollees who are on an application where a new applicant is enrolling in coverage through a special enrollment period. As proposed, this rule would ensure that enrollees who qualify for a special enrollment period or are on an application where an applicant qualifies for a special enrollment period to newly enroll in coverage are not using this special enrollment period to simply switch levels of coverage during the benefit year. This policy would apply to most Exchange enrollees who qualify for a special enrollment period during the benefit year, further protecting issuers from adverse selection. Affected special enrollment periods include special enrollment periods for enrollees who lost minimum essential coverage through the Exchange during the benefit year in accordance with paragraph (d)(1); demonstrated to the Exchange that the QHP into which they have enrolled has violated a material provision of its contract in accordance with paragraph (d)(5); gained access to a new QHP due to a permanent move in accordance with paragraph (d)(7); or were affected by material plan or benefit display errors in accordance with paragraph (d)(12). Enrollees who qualify for the special enrollment periods in paragraphs (d)(4), (d)(9), and (d)(10) would be excluded from this new requirement because the qualifying events that enable them to qualify for these special enrollment periods may also result in an inability to enroll in their desired plan during the annual open enrollment period. In addition, we proposed to exclude the special enrollment period in paragraph (d)(8) for Indians and their dependents from this requirement. We solicited comments on the proposal, and whether other special enrollment periods should be excluded. We also solicited comments on the appropriate transitional period to enable SBEs to build these capacities, or whether the proposals in paragraph (a)(4) should be at the option of the Exchanges. Lastly, we solicited comments on how this proposal would be operationalized in the individual market outside of the Exchanges.

For Exchanges, we are finalizing these provisions largely as proposed, with slight changes to make it clearer that the new paragraph (a)(3) of §155.420 is applicable, in all circumstances, except for the circumstances specified in paragraph (a)(4) (relating to restrictions limiting the plans into which current enrollees may enroll through certain special enrollment periods). Paragraph (a)(3) applies to qualified individuals who are not current enrollees, as well as current enrollees other than current enrollees covered by paragraph (a)(4), such as Exchange enrollees who are eligible for a special enrollment period under paragraph (d)(4), as this special enrollment period is excepted from new paragraph (a)(4)(iii). We are also modifying proposed paragraph (a)(4)(iii) of §155.420 to clarify that this new requirement applies to current enrollees, whether the current enrollee qualifies for a special enrollment period or whether a new qualified individual being added to the current enrollee's QHP qualifies for a special enrollment period, as discussed earlier in this final rule, and to allow these individuals to enroll in an "adjacent" level of coverage, if no other plans are available at their current metal level.

We are also modifying the proposed policy in light of comments received, such that new paragraph (a)(4) will not apply to the individual market outside of the Exchanges because we recognize that requiring issuers outside of the Exchanges to implement this provision would significantly increase issuer burden by requiring the creation of new enrollment systems that would use information that the issuer may not currently possess about the metal level of a consumer's prior coverage. We also recognize that outside of the Exchanges, issuers can perform pre-enrollment verification of special enrollment period eligibility, which mitigates concerns about misuse of special enrollment periods by current enrollees outside of the Exchanges. Accordingly, we are finalizing a new paragraph (b)(2)(iii) in §147.104, rather than the proposed amendments to §147.104(b)(2)(i). Lastly, we are making a technical correction by finalizing new text at §155.725(j)(7), rather than the proposed amendment to §155.725(j)(2)(i), to clearly reflect that §155.420(a)(4) will not apply in the group markets outside of the Exchanges or in the SHOP.

Comment: Many commenters expressed concerns about our proposal to limit current Exchange enrollees' ability to change plans or metal levels in new proposed §155.420(a)(4). Commenters primarily noted that limiting consumer choice with regard to QHP enrollment is prohibited by section 1311(c)(6)(C) of the PPACA and violates the guaranteed issue provision at 42 U.S.C. 300gg-1, in addition to being inconsistent with current industry practice for employer-sponsored coverage, HIPAA, and Medicare Part D. Commenters noted that that the events that qualify these Exchange enrollees for special enrollment periods midyear may also impact the type of coverage they qualify for, the amount of coverage they can afford, and the level of coverage they need. Commenters also observed that special enrollment periods are natural times for households to re- evaluate their healthcare spending. In addition, commenters expressed concerns that this policy would disadvantage consumers who enroll in coverage through the Exchanges during the annual open enrollment period and subsequently experience a qualifying event and want to change their QHP enrollment, as opposed to those who are enrolled in off-Exchange coverage at the beginning of the benefit year and then, upon experiencing a qualifying event, decide to enroll in QHP coverage through the Exchanges. The latter group would be able to view and select among all QHPs for which they are qualified, while the former group would not. For young and healthy consumers, commenters warned that this lack of choice may incentivize them to drop coverage midyear, rather than maintain coverage in a QHP or at a metal level they no longer want. Some commenters requested clarification on the issue that HHS is trying to solve with this proposed policy and requested data to justify implementing these restrictions. One commenter expressed doubt that this policy, if finalized, would be an effective method to protect issuers from gaming and other misuse of special enrollment periods.

In contrast, several commenters supported restricting enrollees' ability to change metal levels during the year, which they believe will increase the integrity of the Exchange markets and improve the risk pool by reducing adverse selection and preventing households from re-evaluating healthcare needs midyear, as opposed to during open enrollment like the rest of the individual market. Several commenters expressed general support for this policy, but requested that HHS permit consumers who qualify for any of these special enrollment periods to be able to change their QHP enrollment to a different QHP at the same metal level or a lower metal level. In addition, one commenter supports this proposal as a short-term strategy to reduce misuse and abuse of special enrollment periods, but would prefer that we move toward verification of eligibility for special enrollment periods for existing Exchange enrollees in the future, and another commenter preferred that the agency require verification of eligibility for special enrollment periods right away.

Response: We understand commenters' concerns about limiting enrollees' choice when they qualify for a special enrollment period during the benefit year and appreciate the fact that households' health coverage needs may change throughout the year. However, we believe putting these restrictions in place is necessary in order to stabilize the Exchanges, which will benefit all Exchange enrollees moving forward. We continue to encourage enrollees to explore all available QHPs during open enrollment and to change plans if another QHP better meets their or their family's needs.

We considered the concerns regarding conflicts with the statute, but believe that limiting enrollees' ability to change

QHPs or metal levels is consistent with the requirements in section 1311(c)(6)(C) of the PPACA directing the Secretary to require Exchanges to establish special enrollment periods as specified in section 9801 of the Code and under circumstances similar to such periods under Part D of title XVIII of the Act, as well as the Secretary's authority under section 2702(b)(3) of the PHS Act to promulgate regulations for the individual market with respect to special enrollment periods for qualifying events under section 603 of the Employee Retirement Income Security Act of 1974. Given that the PPACA itself called for one annual open enrollment period and additional enrollment opportunities only in the case of special circumstances, we believe it is reasonable to interpret the special enrollment period and guaranteed issue provisions of the PPACA in this manner.

Comment: Commenters expressed concerns about our proposal at §155.420(a)(4)(i) to limit the ability of existing enrollees to change QHPs when enrolling a new dependent. Commenters stated that this restriction may negatively affect the healthcare access and health of babies and children, especially if their parents' current coverage is not well suited to their needs, for example, if it does not cover their needed pediatric doctors or medication or other services for a specific health condition.

Several commenters supported restricting the ability of new parents or any applicable existing enrollees to change their QHP enrollment, but many disagreed with placing the same restrictions on new minor dependents, especially babies, for whom the family is unable to anticipate their healthcare needs in advance. Several commenters requested that we establish an exceptions process for babies who have increased healthcare needs that would not be covered under their parents' existing plan. Commenters also noted that changes in household size, which are likely the case for all consumers qualifying for one of the gain a dependent special enrollment periods at §155.420(d)(2)(i), may impact a household's ability to qualify for new, more cost-effective QHPs or to newly qualify for, or qualify for more, financial assistance.

Some commenters requested that in addition to implementing this new restriction on enrollees' ability to change their QHP, HHS clarify that the special enrollment periods at §155.420(d)(2)(i) are only intended for the new dependent and that other members of the household may not enroll in or change coverage through this special enrollment period.

Response: We appreciate the concerns raised by commenters about potential impacts of this policy on new dependents, especially babies and children, and would like to clarify that, under this policy, new dependents could enroll in a new QHP at any metal level, if they enroll in a separate QHP from other existing enrollees. The restrictions on changing QHPs only applies when the new dependent is enrolling in the same QHP with those who are already QHP enrollees. We also remind commenters that the special enrollment period at §155.420(d)(2)(i) as currently written is intended for both those who have gained a dependent or become a dependent through marriage, birth, adoption, placement for adoption, placement in foster care, or through a child support or other court order. Therefore, both the dependent and the individual who gained a dependent are entitled to newly enroll in a QHP, or, if current enrollees, change to a new QHP at the same metal level if the new dependent cannot be added to the existing QHP because of applicable business rules. Alternatively, the dependent can enroll in a new policy at any metal level.

Comment: Commenters raised concerns about §155.420(a)(4)(ii) negatively affecting consumers who, despite newly qualifying for cost-sharing reductions, would prefer to enroll in a QHP at a different metal level and forgo those cost-sharing reductions. Commenters were divided on the anticipated impact of this proposal, with some commenters stating that most enrollees in this situation are likely to already be enrolled in a silver plan or that this is likely the level of coverage they will want given their change in circumstance, so there would be minimal impact of this restriction.

Response: We understand commenters' concerns about limiting the ability of these consumers to change to the QHP metal level that they believe will be most beneficial. However, the rationale behind this particular special enrollment period is to allow individuals newly eligible for cost- sharing reductions to enroll in a plan through which they could receive cost- sharing reductions.

Comment: Commenters supported excluding members of Federally recognized tribes or Alaska Native Claims Settlement Act Corporation Shareholders from the new requirements at §155.420(a)(4)(iii). Several commenters expressed concern about the metal level restrictions in paragraph (a)(4)(iii) if an existing enrollee qualifies for a special enrollment period and there are no other QHPs at their current metal level into which he or she could enroll. Commenters stated that this provision would prevent this consumer from utilizing that special enrollment period.

Response: We agree that members of Federally recognized tribes or Alaska

Native Claims Settlement Act Corporation Shareholders should not be subject to these new requirements and are finalizing their exclusion as proposed. We also agree that, in the event that an enrollee qualifies for a special enrollment period or is adding an individual to his or her existing QHP during the year through a special enrollment period and there are no other QHPs at the enrollee's current metal level into which he or she can enroll, he or she should be permitted to enroll in an adjacent level of coverage. We have amended paragraph (a)(4)(iii) to reflect this flexibility.

Comment: Commenters expressed concern that the complexity of these proposals will lead to consumer confusion, as well as confusion by assisters and others providing enrollment assistance. The level of complexity of these requirements also raised concerns for commenters about SBEs' ability to both build for and comply with these requirements, and the commenters requested that States be given flexibility with respect to implementation. One commenter also questioned how these requirements could be implemented outside of the Exchange, where issuers do not currently receive information about consumers' prior coverage. To that end, commenters noted that these provisions would be burdensome to implement, requiring significant technical builds by Exchanges and stakeholder trainings.

Response: We acknowledge the complexity of these provisions and are taking time to properly plan for their implementation, including developing needed resources for consumers, agents, brokers, Navigators, and other assisters so that they will understand available options. While we encourage SBEs to implement these provisions as quickly as possible, we also appreciate that it will require time for them to make sure that the provisions are implemented correctly. We agree that it would be difficult to implement these requirements outside of the Exchanges, where issuers do not currently receive information about consumers' prior coverage, and therefore are not finalizing our proposal to apply the requirements in new §155.420(a)(4) outside of the individual market Exchanges, and are finalizing revised language in §147.104 to reflect this.

c. Special Enrollment Period Coverage Effective Dates

In the 2018 Payment Notice, HHS finalized paragraph (b)(5) to allow a consumer to request a later coverage effective date than originally assigned if his or her enrollment was delayed due to an eligibility verification and the consumer would be required to pay 2 or more months of retroactive premium in order to effectuate coverage or avoid cancellation. When finalizing this amendment, we did not limit how much later the coverage effective date could be. After further consideration of concerns raised by stakeholders regarding potential adverse selection impacts, we proposed modifying that option and instead allowing consumers to start their coverage no more than 1 month later than their effective date would ordinarily have been, if the special enrollment period verification process delays their enrollment such that they would be required to pay 2 or more months of retroactive premium to effectuate coverage or avoid cancellation. We interpret 2 or more months of retroactive premium to mean that, at the time that the enrollment transaction is sent by the FFE to the issuer, no less than 2 months has elapsed from the date that the consumer's coverage was originally scheduled to begin. As proposed, a consumer who was originally scheduled to begin coverage on March 1, may elect to have coverage start on (and premiums payable for) April 1, if at the end of the document verification process, the enrollment transaction was sent to the issuer at such a time that would require retroactive payment of premiums for March and April. We noted that we do not anticipate that many consumers would be eligible to request a later effective date under this paragraph, as we do not expect the pre-enrollment verification processes to result in such delays. However, we recognized that there may be unforeseen challenges as we implement the verification process and believe it is important to offer this flexibility in the event of such delays. We also noted that we believe the option to have a later effective date could help keep healthier individuals in the market, who otherwise might be deterred by the prospect of paying for 2 or more months of retroactive coverage that they did not use. We solicited comments on this proposal, and the appropriate coverage effective date for these consumers.

We are finalizing this policy as proposed, but are making a technical correction to clarify that these consumers would be required to pay retroactive premiums in order to avoid cancellation in accordance with §155.430(e)(2), as opposed to termination. Additionally, in response to comments and to ensure that there is no conflict or confusion with existing binder payment rules we are revising our existing binder payment regulation in new §155.400(e)(1)(iv) to specify that, in the case of a pended enrollment due to special enrollment period eligibility verification, the consumer's binder payment must consist of the premiums due for all months of retroactive coverage through the first prospective month of coverage consistent with the consumer's coverage start date, as described in §155.420(b)(1), (2) and (3) or, if elected, (b)(5), and that the deadline set by the issuer for making this binder payment must be no earlier than 30 calendar days from the date that the issuer receives the enrollment transaction.

Comment: Commenters were divided in their response to the proposal to modify §155.420(b)(5) to allow consumers whose enrollment was delayed due to verification of their eligibility for special enrollment periods and owe 2 or more months of retroactive premium to push their coverage start date forward 1 month, at the option of the consumer. Some commenters supported this proposal and stated that it balanced the needs of different stakeholders. Other commenters supported this proposal for providing consumer flexibility. They maintained that consumers should not have to pay premiums for several months of retroactive coverage caused by processing delays beyond the consumer's control. Other commenters opposed the proposal because it would limit existing consumer flexibility. They contended that, if verification of special enrollment periods was delayed by more than 2 months, then consumers should have the flexibility to select an appropriate coverage effective date in accordance with the current §155.420(b)(5), and not be limited to a coverage effective date only 1 month later than the date originally assigned. Additional commenters raised concerns about the fact that consumers might be in this situation due to delays at an Exchange and recommended that our policy instead be that if consumers' verification is delayed by 5 or more days (other commenters suggested by 15 or more days) due to delays at an Exchange, then the Exchange should release their pended enrollment, so that they may start using their coverage.

Other commenters opposed the proposal because they stated it could promote adverse selection. They contended that healthy consumers would be incentivized to delay their coverage effective date by 1 month, while sicker consumers would not. They recommended that, if the rule is finalized, consumers should be required to select their coverage effective date at the time of QHP selection. The appropriate coverage effective date should then be sent to the issuer through the consumer's enrollment transaction. In addition, a few commenters recommended that this paragraph be amended to limit this flexibility to delays caused by the Exchanges, as opposed to including consumer delays in submitting documentation.

Several commenters expressed the need for State flexibility in adopting and implementing this proposal. Finally, a few commenters questioned how the proposal would coordinate with a continuous coverage requirement and urged HHS to consider that when crafting future policy around continuous coverage. Specifically, commenters were concerned that delays in verification could result in coverage lapses for which consumers could be penalized if policies requiring continuous coverage or the imposition of a waiting period or premium surcharge were adopted.

Response: We appreciate the variety of perspectives received on this proposal and agree with commenters that this provision strikes a balance of providing consumer flexibility while protecting from adverse selection. We clarify that consumers who qualify for a special enrollment period due to adoption, placement for adoption, placement in foster care, or through a child support or other court order at §155.420(d)(2)(i), are still entitled to the alternative coverage effective date options as described in paragraphs §155.420(b)(2)(i) and (v), at the option of the Exchange. In addition, any SBE conducting a pre-enrollment verification of eligibility for special enrollment periods must also provide this flexibility for consumers. For the FFEs and SBE-FPs, we plan to implement this provision initially through a manual process, and will explore ways to automate such a date shift in the future. SBEs are encouraged to do the same.

d. Tightening Other Special Enrollment Periods

As part of our enhanced verification efforts for special enrollment periods, we proposed to take additional steps to strengthen and streamline the parameters of several existing special enrollment periods and ensure consumers are adhering to existing and new eligibility parameters to further promote continuity of coverage and market stability.

First, in order to ensure that a special enrollment period for loss of minimum essential coverage in paragraph (d)(1) is not granted in cases where an individual was terminated for non- payment of premium, as described in paragraph (e)(1), we proposed that FFE (and SBE–FPs) will permit the issuer to reject an enrollment for which the issuer has a record of termination due to non- payment of premiums by the individual, unless the individual fulfills obligations for premiums due for previous coverage, consistent with the guaranteed availability approach discussed in the preamble of this final rule for §147.104. We noted that we believe that verifying that consumers are not attempting to enroll in coverage through the special enrollment period for loss of minimum essential coverage when the reason for their loss of coverage is due to non-payment of premiums is an important measure to prevent instances of gaming related to individuals only paying premiums and maintaining coverage for months in which they seek services.

Further, HHS intends to explore options for verifying that a consumer's coverage was not terminated due to non- payment of premiums for coverage within the FFEs as a precursor for being eligible for the loss of minimum essential coverage special enrollment period. We proposed to allow Exchanges to collect and store information from issuers about whether consumers have been terminated from Exchange coverage due to nonpayment of premiums, so that the Exchange may automatically prevent these consumers from qualifying for the special enrollment period due to a loss of minimum essential coverage, if the consumer attempts to renew his or her Exchange coverage within 60 days of being terminated. We noted that we are focused on the 60 days following termination because if the consumer attempts to renew his or her Exchange coverage more than 60 days after being terminated due to nonpayment of premiums, the Exchange would continue to find the consumer ineligible for a special enrollment period because the loss of minimum essential coverage would be more than 60 days prior, and therefore the individual would not be eligible for the loss of minimum essential coverage special enrollment period.

We are finalizing these provisions as proposed, and we additionally clarify that the FFE (and SBE-FPs) will permit the issuers in the same controlled group as the issuer that has a record of termination due to non-payment of premiums to refuse to effectuate new coverage, unless the individual pays sufficient premiums to fulfill his or her obligations for past-due premiums and to make the required binder payment, consistent with the guaranteed availability approach discussed in the preamble for §147.104, and the binder payment requirements in §155.400(e).

Comment: Commenters had mixed reactions to our proposals to allow issuers to reject enrollments from consumers previously terminated from coverage due to nonpayment of premiums, and our proposal to allow the FFE to store this information from issuers in order to prevent these consumers from qualifying for a special enrollment due to loss of minimum essential coverage due to termination for nonpayment of premiums.

Commenters in support of these proposals stated that they are necessary to prevent misuse of the special enrollment period for loss of minimum essential coverage. Some stated that the proposals help support continuous coverage by ensuring that consumers do not stop paying their premiums in order to be terminated from coverage for a portion of the year only to re-enroll in coverage when health needs arise. Encouraging both proper use of special enrollment periods and continuous coverage, commenters stated, will improve the risk pool moving forward.

Commenters opposing these proposals cautioned that there are legitimate reasons why consumers might stop paying their premiums midyear that are unrelated to a desire to game the system, such as a reduction in household income, other pressing needs that affect household finances, or technical issues in making premium payments. In addition, some commenters observed that some consumers who want to terminate their coverage experience difficulty or confusion over how to end it, resulting in termination due to nonpayment of premiums. Commenters expressed concern that giving issuers the authority to reject enrollments received through the Exchange is a slippery slope towards allowing issuers to make eligibility determinations for coverage, and asked that HHS ensure that Exchanges continue to make eligibility determinations. Finally, commenters expressed concern that HHS may be making it too difficult for consumers to enroll in coverage with these proposals, leading to consumers getting caught in a cycle of being uninsurable.

Response: We appreciate commenters' concerns about our proposals to prevent consumers who were terminated from coverage due to nonpayment of premium from enrolling in coverage midyear through a special enrollment period due to loss of minimum essential coverage, but believe that these provisions are an important step to ensuring that consumers are not obtaining Exchange coverage through special enrollment periods only when healthcare needs arise. We believe that it is important for consumers to maintain continuous coverage both as protection against unforeseen health needs and to create stability in the individual market, and therefore are finalizing these provisions as proposed, with a modification to reflect the revised interpretation of guaranteed availability discussed in the preamble for §147.104.

Second, in response to concerns that consumers are opting not to enroll in QHP coverage during the annual open enrollment period and are instead newly enrolling in coverage during the benefit year through the special enrollment period for marriage, we proposed to add new paragraph

(d)(2)(i)(A) to require that, if consumers are newly enrolling in QHP coverage through the Exchange through the special enrollment period for marriage, at least one spouse must demonstrate having had minimum essential coverage as described in 26 CFR 1.5000A-1(b) for 1 or more days during the 60 days preceding the date of marriage. However, we noted that we recognize that individuals who were previously living in a foreign country or in a U.S. territory may not have had access to coverage that is considered minimum essential coverage in accordance with 26 CFR 1.5000A-1(b) prior to moving to the U.S. Therefore, we proposed new paragraph (a)(5), to allow that, when consumers are newly enrolling in coverage during the benefit year through the special enrollment period for marriage, at least one spouse must either demonstrate that they had minimum essential coverage or that they lived in a foreign country or in a U.S. territory for 1 or more days during the 60 days preceding the date of the marriage. We proposed this change for the individual market only.

We are finalizing this provision for the individual market as proposed, with minor modifications to §155.420(a)(5) to: (1) Clarify that by those living outside of the U.S, we mean those living in a foreign country; and (2) exempt Indians, as defined by section 4 of the Indian Health Care Improvement Act, from this requirement due to the fact that the Indian Health Service has not been designated as minimum essential coverage.

Comment: Some commenters supported the proposal to add a new prior coverage requirement for at least one spouse applying for coverage through the special enrollment period for marriage at §155.420(d)(2)(i)(A) because they believed this new requirement will deter abuse and adverse risk selection and is similar to current special enrollment period eligibility processes for small group plans. Commenters stated that this requirement supports continuous coverage and should also be extended to all applicable special enrollment periods. One commenter requested that it be extended to both spouses. Commenters requested that any prior coverage standards and verification methods be standardized across markets.

However, many commenters opposed this proposal and expressed concern that requiring a prior coverage requirement for the special enrollment period for marriage is prohibited by section 1311(c)(6)(C) of the PPACA and violates guaranteed issue provisions at 42 U.S.C. 300gg-1, in addition to being inconsistent with current industry practice for employer sponsored coverage, HIPAA, and Medicare Part D. Commenters stated that the existing individual shared responsibility provision is a sufficient deterrent to prevent these consumers from avoiding coverage prior to marriage, if otherwise eligible. Of particular concern to these commenters was that one or both spouses may have been ineligible for affordable coverage prior to marriage due to the gap in insurance affordability program eligibility for individuals under the poverty line in States that did not expand their Medicaid program.

Some commenters also expressed concern that this requirement and any onerous verification process will discourage participation of newly married individuals, who are more likely to be part of the young and healthy population needed to balance the risk pool. Commenters also expressed concern that consumers who qualify for this special enrollment period may have had prior coverage but may not have documentation to submit due to the elimination of the prior HIPAA requirement for issuers and health plans to send enrollees certificates of credible coverage, and requested that, in the event that this provision is finalized, that this requirement be reinstated.

In addition, commenters requested that SBEs be given flexibility on the effective date of this provision, recognizing the resources needed to comply, and to allow for adequate time for implementation.

Response: We agree with comments noting the potential for this provision to reduce adverse selection and promote continuous coverage. The proposed rule aims to stabilize the individual market, such that coverage will be more accessible and affordable for all potential enrollees.

We considered the concerns regarding conflicts with the statute, but believe that the additional requirement for marriage special enrollment period eligibility is consistent with the requirement in section 1311(c)(6)(C) of the PPACA directing the Secretary to require Exchanges to establish special enrollment periods as specified in section 9801 of the Code and under circumstances similar to such periods under Part D of title XVIII of the Act and the Secretary's authority under section 2702(b)(3) of the PHS Act to promulgate regulations for the individual market with respect to special enrollment periods for qualifying events under section 603 of the Employee Retirement Income Security Act of 1974. The PPACA itself called for one annual open enrollment period and additional opportunities for enrollment only in the case of special circumstances. Section 155.420(d) provides each of the special enrollment periods required by section 1311(c)(6)(C) of the PPACA and section 2702(b)(3) of the PHS Act. Section 1321(a) of the PPACA grants the Secretary broad discretion to issue regulations setting standards with respect to the operation of the Exchange program and other requirements the Secretary determines are appropriate to support its viability. Given that there is nothing in section 1311(c)(6)(C) of the PPACA that otherwise limits the Secretary's broad discretion under section 1321(a) of the PPACA, we believe we may place reasonable limits on access to special enrollment periods that promote the overall goal of the PPACA to ensure continuous health coverage and the viability of Exchanges.

We are also sensitive to commenter concerns regarding the coverage gap that might prevent some consumers from having access to affordable coverage prior to marriage. However, if the married couple's combined income makes them newly eligible for APTC then that couple would be able to qualify for the special enrollment period for consumers in this situation at §155.420(d)(6)(iv), and would not need to enroll through the marriage special enrollment period.

We appreciate commenters' concerns that adding a prior coverage requirement to the marriage special enrollment period would discourage enrollment by this population, but we believe that this requirement is important to ensure that previously uninsured individuals do not negatively impact the risk pool. In response to the comments regarding certificates of credible coverage, we note that per sections 1502 and 1514 of the PPACA and section 6055 of the Code, enrollees have proof of previous year health coverage via their tax statements that may help in certain circumstances. We also note that the FFEs and SBE-FPs will accept other types of documentation from consumers to verify their prior coverage, including letters from insurers, employers, and government health programs. We will also exercise reasonable flexibility with respect to the documentation required under this policy.

While we are not adjusting the effective date of the regulation, we understand that the prior coverage requirement may require system changes that take additional time for some SBEs and expect that Exchanges will implement the requirement as soon as technically feasible.

Comment: Commenters requested that members of Federally recognized tribes and Alaska Claims Settlement Act Corporation Shareholders be excluded from this requirement because the Indian Health Service, a major provider of healthcare services for members of Federally recognized tribes, is not designated as minimum essential coverage, thus individuals moving off of tribal land after a marriage and seeking to enroll in Exchange coverage will not be able to prove prior coverage.

Response: We agree with commenters that members of Federally recognized tribes and Alaska Claims Settlement Act Corporation Shareholders should be excluded from this prior coverage requirement, in addition to the prior coverage requirement for permanent move at §155.420(d)(7), and finalize a modification to our proposed regulation at §155.420(a)(5) accordingly.

To streamline our regulations regarding special enrollment periods that require consumers to demonstrate prior coverage, we proposed to add new paragraph (a)(5) to clarify that qualified individuals who are required to demonstrate prior coverage can either demonstrate that they had minimum essential coverage as described in 26 CFR 1.5000A-1(b) for 1 or more days during the 60 days preceding the date of the qualifying event or that they lived in a foreign country or in a U.S. territory for 1 or more days during the 60 days preceding the date of the qualifying event. Paragraph (a)(5) would apply to paragraph (d)(2)(i)(A) for marriage (discussed above) and paragraph (d)(7)(i) for permanent move and paragraph (a)(5) would replace current paragraph (d)(7)(ii).

We did not receive comment on this proposal and are finalizing it as proposed, with minor modifications: (1) To clarify that by those living outside of the U.S. we mean those living in a foreign country; and (2) to exempt Indians, as defined by section 4 of the Indian Health Care Improvement Act, from this requirement due to the fact that the Indian Health Service is not designated as minimum essential coverage. Additionally, the finalized amendments to §155.725(j) include a change to the proposed text to reflect that the new prior coverage requirement for the marriage special enrollment period under §155.420(d)(2) does not apply outside of the individual market. The proposed rule had incorrectly cross- referenced §155.420(a)(5), which describes how the prior coverage requirement may be satisfied. We had not intended in the proposed rule to prevent individuals applying for special enrollment periods under §155.420(d)(7) in the SHOP from satisfying the prior coverage requirement as specified under §155.420(a)(5). We note that §155.420(a)(5) is already incorporated through the cross-references to revised §155.420(d) in §155.725(j)(2)(i). Similarly, we note that we are finalizing that §155.420(a)(5), specifying how an individual can demonstrate prior coverage, applies in the individual market outside of the Exchange, but determined that the proposed change to §147.104(b)(2)(i), which would have specified this, is not necessary because §155.420(a)(5) is already incorporated through the cross-reference to revised §155.420(d) in §147.104(b)(2).

We acknowledge that the proposed rule included changes for special enrollment periods in the individual market that differ from the rules regarding special enrollment periods in the group market. For example, the proposed rule included changes that would require consumers to demonstrate prior coverage to qualify for the special enrollment period for marriage in proposed paragraph (d)(2)(i)(A) and would generally limit plan selection to the same plan or level of coverage when an enrollee qualifies for a special enrollment period during the benefit year in proposed paragraph (a)(4). However, we noted that we believe that the differences in the markets—and the impacts of those differences on the risk pool—warrant an approach in the individual market that diverges from long-standing rules and norms in the group market. Employer-sponsored coverage is generally a more stable risk pool and less susceptible to gaming because the coverage is tied to employment and often substantially subsidized by the employer. Thus, we noted that we believe taking an approach in the individual market that imposes tighter restrictions on special enrollment periods and the ability to change plans for current enrollees better addresses the unique challenges faced in the individual market. We also noted that this approach is consistent with the requirement in section 1311(c)(6)(C) of the PPACA directing the Secretary to require Exchanges to establish special enrollment periods as specified in section 9801 of the Code and under circumstances similar to such periods under Part D of title XVIII of the Act and the Secretary's authority under section 2702(b)(3) of the PHS Act to promulgate regulations for the individual market with respect to special enrollment periods for qualifying events under section 603 of the Employee Retirement Income Security Act of 1974. We interpret section 1311 of the PPACA and section 2702 of the PHS Act to require the Secretary to implement special enrollment periods with the same triggering events as in the group market, but to provide the Secretary with flexibility in the specific parameters as to how those special enrollment periods are implemented in the individual market, due to the unique dynamics of the individual market.

Third, we proposed to expand the verification requirements related to the special enrollment period for a permanent move in paragraph (d)(7). This special enrollment period is only available to a qualified individual or enrollee who has gained access to new QHPs as a result of a permanent move *and* had coverage for 1 or more days in the 60 days preceding the move, unless he or she is moving to the U.S. from a foreign country or a U.S. territory. (Following finalization of the changes discussed above to paragraph (a)(5), individuals will also be exempt from demonstrating prior coverage if they demonstrate they are Indians.) Currently, we require documentation to show a move occurred, and accept an attestation regarding having had prior coverage or moving from a foreign country or a U.S. territory. To ensure that consumers meet all the requirements for this special enrollment period, we proposed to require that new applicants applying for coverage through this special enrollment period submit acceptable documentation to the FFEs and SBE-FPs to prove both their move and evidence of prior coverage, if applicable, through the pre-enrollment verification process.

We are finalizing this provision as proposed and intend to release guidance on what documentation would be acceptable.

Comment: Comments were mixed regarding our proposal to expand the verification requirements for individuals seeking a permanent move special enrollment period. Commenters who supported this proposal stated that requiring and verifying prior coverage is necessary to prevent misuse and abuse of this special enrollment period, which will protect the risk pool.

Commenters who opposed this proposal expressed concerns that some individuals may have been ineligible for affordable coverage where they were previously living or may experience barriers to providing proof of prior coverage. Commenters expressed concerns about consumer capacity to procure needed documents, especially if the consumer was formerly enrolled in Medicaid. Others expressed specific concerns about the ability of vulnerable low-income workers who often move for work to produce documentation, since their employers often do not provide documentation and insurance companies are no longer required to do so via certificates of credible coverage.

In addition, several commenters supported using electronic methods to verify both prior coverage and the permanent move, when able, to decrease the burden on consumers.

Response: We appreciate commenters' input on the merits and drawbacks of requiring consumers to submit evidence of prior coverage or evidence that they are exempt from the requirement to show prior coverage. Although we agree that some consumers may have legitimate reasons for not obtaining coverage prior to their move, we established in prior rulemaking that prior coverage is generally a requirement to qualify for the permanent move special enrollment period, and we did not propose to change this requirement in the proposed rule. We agree with those commenters who believed that the proposed additional verification steps were necessary to prevent abuse and misuse of this special enrollment period, and therefore, we will finalize our proposal to verify prior coverage for this special enrollment period, when applicable. As mentioned earlier in this section, we will also exercise reasonable flexibility with respect to the documentation required under this policy.

We agree with comments regarding use of electronic verification where available and are investigating our ability to expand our use of electronic verification and encourage SBEs to do the same. We also clarify that these changes only apply in the individual market.

Fourth, for the remainder of 2017 and for future plan years, we proposed to significantly limit the use of the exceptional circumstances special enrollment period described in paragraph (d)(9). In previous years, this special enrollment period has been used to address eligibility or enrollment issues that affected large cohorts of individuals where they had made reasonable efforts to enroll but were hindered by outside events. For example, in past years, the FFEs have offered exceptional circumstances special enrollment periods to groups of consumers who were enrolled in coverage that they believed was minimum essential coverage at the time of enrollment, but was not. We proposed to apply a more rigorous test for future uses of the exceptional circumstances special enrollment period, including requiring supporting documentation where practicable, under which we would only grant this special enrollment period if provided with sufficient evidence to conclude that the consumer's situation was highly exceptional and in instances where it is verifiable that consumers were directly impacted by the circumstance, as practicable. We would provide guidance on examples of situations that we believe meet this more rigorous text and what corresponding documentation consumers would be required to provide, if requested by the FFE.

We are finalizing this provision as proposed.

Comment: We received comments both supporting and opposing our proposal to limit the use of the special enrollment period for exceptional circumstances. One commenter supported this proposal because of a belief that this special enrollment should only be used for truly exceptional circumstances and should not be used to provide a pathway to coverage for large categories of consumers.

Commenters opposing the proposal generally expressed concern that Exchanges have already imposed sufficient constraints with regard to granting eligibility for this special enrollment period and expressed concern that this proposal would prevent eligible consumers experiencing situations outside of their control from enrolling in coverage. Commenters also questioned whether HHS would be able to adequately establish guidelines for this special enrollment period because it is used for situations that are unanticipated and unpredictable. Several commenters requested that HHS publish more guidance either in the final rule or guidance as to what qualifies as an exceptional circumstance for the purposes of this special enrollment period.

A few commenters noted the importance of allowing SBEs flexibility to determine what constitutes an exceptional circumstance.

Response: The exceptional circumstances special enrollment period provides an important avenue to coverage for consumers who experience or are affected by unanticipated events, often outside of their control. We agree that this special enrollment period should be granted as consistently as possible based on established criteria, while still allowing enough flexibility to account for the inherent unpredictability of exceptional circumstances. Currently, the vast majority of exceptional circumstances special enrollment periods granted through the FFEs are reviewed in detail by HHS staff and evaluated based on standardized protocols. We believe this process balances the need for standardization and flexibility while ensuring that claims of exceptional circumstances can be verified. HHS expects to continue using this process as it applies a more rigorous test for future uses of the exceptional circumstances special enrollment period. We believe SBEs should retain the flexibility to determine what constitutes an exceptional circumstance, but we urge them to establish a similar process to grant such special enrollment periods consistently and, to help in this effort, as we mentioned in the proposed rule, we expect to provide additional guidance on what constitutes an exceptional circumstance for the purposes of qualifying for this special enrollment period and clarify that this change only applies to the individual market.

Previously, the Exchanges have, at times, offered special enrollment periods for a variety of circumstances related to errors that occurred more frequently in the early years of operations. As the Exchanges continue to mature, HHS has previously evaluated, and will continue to evaluate, these existing special enrollment periods to determine their continued utility and necessity. For the purposes of clarity and in response to confusion by stakeholders about whether certain of these special enrollment periods previously made available through guidance are still available to consumers, we proposed to formalize previous guidance[55] from HHS that the following special enrollment periods are no longer available:

- Consumers who enrolled with APTC that is too large because of a redundant or duplicate policy;
- Consumers who were affected by a temporary error in the treatment of Social Security Income for tax dependents;
- Lawfully present non-citizens that were affected by a temporary error in
- the determination of their eligibility for APTC;
- Lawfully present non-citizens with incomes below 100 percent of Federal Poverty Level (FPL) who experienced certain processing delays; and
- Consumers who were eligible for or enrolled in COBRA and not sufficiently informed about their coverage options.
- We are finalizing this provision as proposed.

Comment: A few commenters expressed concern about our proposal to codify the elimination of several special enrollment periods that were eliminated through prior guidance due to fear that we are cutting off the availability of special enrollment periods to vulnerable populations that need a pathway to coverage.

Response: The special enrollment periods listed for elimination in this rule have not been available to consumers since 2016; they were originally eliminated in subregulatory guidance because all consumers in the situations described had already been provided with a pathway to coverage. Codifying the elimination of these special enrollment periods will not affect vulnerable consumers' ability to access coverage in the future.

4. Continuous Coverage

Because of the challenges in the individual market related to adverse selection, HHS believes it is especially important in this market to adopt policies that promote continuous enrollment in health coverage and to encourage individuals to enroll and remain in coverage for the full year.

While the provisions in this rule relating to guaranteed availability, the annual open enrollment period, and special enrollment periods encourage individuals to maintain coverage throughout the year, we noted in the proposed rule that we are also actively exploring additional policies in the individual market that would promote continuous coverage and sought input on which policies would effectively do so, consistent with existing legal authorities. For example, with respect to special enrollment periods that require evidence of prior coverage, we are considering policies for the individual market that would require that individuals show evidence of prior coverage for a longer "look back" period. Individuals could be required to provide proof of prior coverage for 6 to 12 months, except that an individual with a small gap in coverage (such as up to 60 days), could be considered to have had prior coverage. Alternatively, for individuals who are not able to provide evidence of prior coverage during such a look back period, an exception could allow them to enroll in coverage if they otherwise qualify for a special enrollment period, but impose a waiting period of at least 90 days before effectuating enrollment, or assess a late enrollment penalty. These policies could encourage individuals to maintain coverage throughout the year, thus promoting continuous coverage.

HHS is also interested in whether policies are needed for the individual market similar to those that existed under HIPAA, which in the group market required maintenance of continuous, creditable coverage without a 63-day break if individuals wished to avoid the pre-existing condition exclusions, and allowed waiting periods to be imposed under certain circumstances. Although the HIPAA rules did not require that individuals maintain coverage, the rules were designed to provide an important incentive for individuals to enroll in coverage for the full year, not just when in need of healthcare services; reduce adverse selection; and help prevent premiums from climbing to levels that would keep most healthy individuals from purchasing coverage.

We are interested in policies that not only encourage uninsured individuals to enroll in coverage during the open enrollment period, but also encourage those with coverage to maintain continuous coverage throughout the year.

We solicited comments on additional policies that would promote continuous coverage, but did not propose any of the policies described in this section III.B.3. of this final rule. The following is a summary of the public comments received on the discussed continuous coverage policies and our responses:

Comment: A minority of commenters, primarily issuers, supported the policies discussed in the proposed rule, or the general concept of policies to promote continuous coverage. Many of these commenters emphasized the need for policies like continuous coverage requirements, waiting periods or late enrollment penalties, if the individual shared responsibility provision is eliminated. These commenters recommended imposing longer look- back periods of varying lengths for special enrollment periods; a few recommended late enrollment surcharges of specific amounts (for example, 150 percent, lasting for at least 18 months); and one commenter expressed a preference for premium penalties over making prior coverage an eligibility requirement for special enrollment periods. Several of these commenters cautioned HHS against re-introducing waiting periods, noting the operational burden, consumer harm, or perceived limited effectiveness as compared to other penalties for having a coverage lapse. Several commenters noted the importance of clearly communicating continuous coverage requirements to consumers.

Some commenters believed continuous coverage policies should apply during open enrollment. One commenter recommended that if a continuous coverage policy were adopted that applied only to special enrollment periods, an exemption from the look-back period should be provided to anyone who enrolled during the most recent open enrollment period. That commenter also believed that the longer the look-back period is, the stronger the incentive to remain insured and the less opportunity to game the system; and commented that the discussed policies could result in reduced usage of special enrollment periods and higher out-of- pocket costs for consumers. Some commenters opposed applying continuous coverage requirements to special enrollment periods. A few commenters specifically urged HHS to exempt the monthly special enrollment period for Indians and their dependents from any continuous coverage requirements. Some commenters observed that some of the changes being finalized in this rule, particularly those related to verification of eligibility for special enrollment periods, could result in more people experiencing coverage lapses.

The majority of commenters opposed the adoption of the continuous coverage policies discussed in this section. Many commenters believed the discussed policies would deter individuals from purchasing coverage in the individual market, would have a negative impact on the risk pool, or increase premiums. Many commenters urged HHS not to adopt policies that would penalize people who have coverage lapses for legitimate reasons. Commenters questioned the premise that coverage lapses were primarily due to gaming behavior. Commenters observed that people often experience coverage gaps for reasons unrelated to gaming behavior, such as financial difficulties paying their premiums, challenges associated with mental or chronic illnesses, job loss, changes in family circumstances (for example, death, divorce or moves), mix-ups with insurance companies or the Exchanges, lack of awareness about the individual shared responsibility provision, and losing APTC. Many of these commenters suggested that the continuous coverage policies discussed in the proposed rule are unlikely to encourage these individuals to maintain coverage, particularly those who are healthy and leaving for economic reasons. Some commenters recommended exceptions be included in any adopted continuous coverage policies to account for individuals who have legitimate reasons not to maintain coverage, or who have received an exemption from the individual shared responsibility provision. Some commenters observed that the people most likely to have gaps in coverage are also the least likely to be able to pay higher premiums, and could thus be locked out of the market after a coverage lapse. Some commenters predicted such policies would increase the uninsured rate. Commenters urged HHS not to adopt policies that would make insurance less affordable.

Many commenters expressed concern that the continuous coverage policies discussed in the proposed rule would hurt consumers, particularly vulnerable populations, including low- and middle-income individuals; seasonal or migratory workers; and individuals with chronic diseases, disabilities, or other pre-existing conditions. Many commenters believed policies that include longer look-back periods, waiting periods, late enrollment penalties, or HIPAA-style rules could disrupt patients' care or cause people to delay or go without care, resulting in increased costs in the future and worse health outcomes. One commenter raised concerns that issuers could game continuous coverage requirements to avoid covering sicker individuals. One commenter also expressed concern that such policies could result in other unintended consequences like increased crime or homelessness. Many commenters were concerned that HHS's interest in policies promoting continuous coverage presaged an end to the prohibitions against pre-existing condition exclusions, medical underwriting, or rescissions (except in limited circumstances).

Some commenters expressed a belief that such policies are immoral. Many commenters stated it was unfair to penalize people once they obtain coverage, or believed it was unfair to apply both the individual shared responsibility provision and penalties associated with continuous coverage requirements.

One commenter noted that it believes HHS has significant authority to impose continuous coverage requirements on all special enrollment periods, although that commenter also recommended exempting several special enrollment periods from continuous coverage requirements. Another commenter noted that they believed current law precludes imposing continuous coverage requirements during open enrollment periods, but not for special enrollment periods. However, many commenters stated that the discussed policies, and pre-existing condition exclusions, were counter to the PPACA's guaranteed availability protections, and that assessing a late enrollment penalty or surcharge was also counter to the requirements regarding rating variations.

Commenters raised concerns related to applying continuous coverage requirements in the individual market, including a concern about applying rules similar to the HIPAA rules outside of the employment context, and a concern about adopting continuous coverage requirements in the individual market that differ from rules for other markets. One commenter strongly opposed requiring SBEs to adopt continuous coverage policies.

Many commenters believed that the individual shared responsibility provision promotes continuous coverage better than the policies discussed in the proposed rule. Some recommended increasing the amount of the individual shared responsibility payment. A few commenters encouraged the Administration to communicate that it intended to enforce the individual shared responsibility provision as a way to stabilize the individual market. Some commenters recommended helping people understand their responsibility under the individual shared responsibility provision as a means to promote continuous coverage. Some commenters provided suggestions for alternative approaches to promote continuous coverage, including minimizing barriers to enrollment, providing more support to people as they enroll, ensuring plans provide adequate value to consumers, making plans more affordable, increasing subsidies, and creating incentives for multi-year enrollments. One commenter recommended enrollees be contractually bound to pay premiums for a full year, with insurers having a mechanism to recover unpaid premiums. Multiple commenters recommended a form of universal healthcare as a way to achieve continuous coverage.

Response: We thank commenters for their input. We continue to explore policies that would promote continuous coverage and that are within HHS's legal authority, and will not take action in this final rule.

5. Enrollment Periods Under SHOP

Because the proposed changes to restrict enrollment options though special enrollment periods for current enrollees and to require a demonstration of prior coverage in order to qualify for the marriage special enrollment period were proposed for special enrollment periods in the individual market only, we proposed to amend §155.725(j)(2)(i) to specify that §155.420(a)(3) through (5) do not apply to special enrollment periods under the Small Business Health Options Program (SHOP). We are finalizing the proposal that the change to restrict enrollment options though special enrollment periods for current enrollees in §155.420(a)(4) and the change to require a demonstration of prior coverage in order to qualify for the marriage special enrollment period these paragraphs do not apply to special enrollment periods under SHOP. However, instead of finalizing the proposed amendment to §155.725(j)(2)(i), we are finalizing a new §155.725(j)(7). This change more clearly reflects that §155.420(a)(4) and the requirement to demonstrate prior coverage to qualify for the marriage special enrollment period do not apply to the SHOP. We note that under the finalized language, §155.420(a)(5) would be applicable to the SHOP. Although the requirement to show prior coverage is not applicable in the SHOP for the marriage special enrollment period, it is applicable for the permanent move special enrollment period under §155.420(d)(7). We had not intended the proposed rule to prevent individuals applying for special enrollment periods under §155.420(d)(7) in the SHOP from satisfying the prior coverage requirement as specified under §155.420(a)(5). A more detailed discussion of the proposed and finalized changes in §155.420(a) is provided in section III.B.3. of this final rule.

The following is a summary of the public comments received on the enrollment periods under the SHOP proposed provisions and our responses:

Comment: Commenters expressed concern about applying different rules for special enrollment periods in the small group and individual markets, noting the potential for confusion among consumers or assisters, and operational challenges; or questioning the need for different rules. One commenter opposed creating a different set of special enrollment period rules between the individual and small group markets because the commenter's State has a merged market such that its qualified health plans are offered in both the individual and small group markets. Some commenters supported not applying the proposed changes to special enrollment periods to the SHOP, and one requested clarification that the changes also not apply to the small group in the off-Exchange market.

Response: We appreciate the comments. We note that there are other rules relating to special enrollment periods where the rules differ for the individual Exchanges and the SHOPs. The finalized rules regarding special enrollment periods in §155.420(a)(4) and (d)(2)(i)(A) do not apply to the small group market.

6. Exchange Functions: Certification of Qualified Health Plans (Part 155, Subpart K)

In light of the need for issuers to make modifications to their products and applications to accommodate the changes finalized in this rule, we are concurrently issuing separate guidance to update the QHP certification calendar and the rate review submission deadlines to give additional time for issuers to develop, and States to review, form and rate filings for the 2018 plan year that reflect these changes.[56]

C. Part 156 – Health Insurance Issuer Standards Under the Patient Protection and Affordable Care Act, Including Standards Related to Exchanges

1. Levels of Coverage (Actuarial Value) (§156.140)

Section 2707(a) of the PHS Act and section 1302 of the PPACA direct issuers of non-grandfathered individual and small group health insurance plans, including QHPs, to ensure that these plans adhere to the levels of coverage specified in section 1302(d)(1) of the PPACA. A plan's coverage level, or AV, is determined based on its coverage of the EHB for a standard population. Section 1302(d)(1) of the PPACA requires a bronze plan to have an AV of 60 percent, a silver plan to have an AV of 70 percent, a gold plan to have an AV of 80 percent, and a platinum plan to have an AV of 90 percent. Section 1302(d)(2) of the PPACA directs the Secretary to issue regulations on the calculation of AV and its application to the levels of coverage. Section 1302(d)(3) of the PPACA authorizes the Secretary to develop guidelines to provide for a de minimis variation in the actuarial valuations used in determining the level of coverage of a plan to account for differences in actuarial estimates.

As stated in the proposed rule, we believe that further flexibility is needed for the AV de minimis range for metal levels to help issuers design new plans for future plan years, thereby promoting competition in the market. In addition, we noted that we believe that changing the de minimis range will allow more plans to keep their cost sharing the same from year to year. More specifically, we noted that as established at §156.135(a), to calculate the AV of a health plan, the issuer must use the AV Calculator developed and made available by HHS for the given benefit year, and that we made several key updates to the AV Calculator for 2018. Due to the scope and number of these updates in the 2018 AV Calculator, the impact on current plans' AVs will vary. Therefore, we proposed to amend the definition of de minimis included in §156.140(c), to a variation of ¥4/+2 percentage points, rather than +/¥ 2 percentage points for all non-grandfathered individual and small group market plans (other than bronze plans meeting certain conditions) that are required to comply with AV. As proposed, for example, a silver plan could have an AV between 66 and 72 percent. We believe a broader de minimis range will provide additional flexibility for issuers to make adjustments to their plans within the same metal level.

While we proposed to modify the de minimis range for the metal level plans (bronze, silver, gold, and platinum), we did not propose to modify the de minimis range for the silver plan variations (the plans with an AV of 73, 87 and 94 percent) under §§156.400 and 156.420. The de minimis variation for a silver plan variation of a single percentage point would still apply. In the Actuarial Value and Cost-Sharing Reductions Bulletin (2012 Bulletin) we issued on February 24, 2012,[57] we explained why we did not intend to require issuers to offer a cost-sharing reduction (CSR) silver plan variation with an AV of 70 percent. However, we proposed to consider whether the ability for an issuer to offer a standard silver plan at an AV of 66 percent would require a silver plan variation to be offered at an AV of 70 percent or would require some other mechanism to provide for CSR silver plan variations for eligible individuals with household incomes that are more than 250 percent but not more than 400 percent of the FPL.

We proposed to maintain the bronze plan de minimis range policy finalized in the 2018 Payment Notice at §156.140(c) with one modification.

We proposed to change the de minimis range for the expanded bronze plans from ¥2/+5 percentage points to ¥4/+5 percentage points to align with the proposed policy. Therefore, for those bronze plans that either cover and pay for at least one major service, other than preventive services, before the deductible or meet the requirements to be a high deductible health plan within the meaning of 26 U.S.C. 223(c)(2), we proposed the allowable variation in AV would be ¥4 percentage points and +5 percentage points.[58]

We solicited comments on the proposal, including on the appropriate de minimis values for metal level plans and silver plan variations, and on whether those values should differ when increasing or decreasing AV. We proposed the policy for 2018, but we also considered proposing that the change be effective for the 2019 plan year. We noted that, if finalized for 2018, we would update the 2018 AV Calculator in accordance with this policy.

We are finalizing the policy as proposed and are adding regulation text to reflect that the policy applies to plan years beginning on or after January 1, 2018. The following is a summary of the public comments received on the levels of coverage (actuarial value) (§156.140) proposed provisions and our responses:

Comment: Some commenters supported the proposed policy as generally increasing issuer flexibility by allowing issuers to offer more innovative plans, to assist with premium impact and to stabilize the market. Others supported the policy for similar reasoning, but recommended a different range or combination, such as +/¥4 percent, as AVs typically go up each year (and not down). Other commenters did not support the proposed range, wanting to keep the current range to ensure consumers can meaningfully compare plan designs. Some commenters stated that the proposed de minimis range was unlawful under section 1302(d)(3) of the PPACA as the de minimis range is to account for differences in actuarial estimates only and not for the reasoning provided in the proposed rule. Some commenters were concerned that the distinction, transparency, and variation between and within metal levels would create consumer confusion and could lead to enrollment issues, with some commenters particularly concerned about the proposed 1 percent difference between bronze and silver levels of coverage and the distinction between those metal levels. A commenter also noted that the policy would allow plan designs that are simultaneously compliant with bronze and silver metal tiers in the Final 2018 AV Calculator (due to the induced demand between metal levels). Other commenters wanted to ensure State AV-related flexibility. Some commenters wanted HHS to engage with stakeholders to consider the impact of the proposal before finalizing the policy. Commenters generally supported retaining the current de minimis range for the CSR silver plan variations.

Response: As discussed in the proposed rule, the health and competitiveness of the Exchanges, as well as the individual and small group markets in general, have recently been threatened by issuer exit and increasing rates in many geographic areas. Therefore, while we recognize the importance of consumers being able to compare plan designs, we are committed to providing issuers increased AV flexibility to improve the health and competitiveness of the markets. For these reasons, we believe that a de minimis range of ¥4/+2 percentage points provides the flexibility necessary for issuers to design new plans while ensuring comparability of plans within each metal level. Through our authority under section 1302(d)(3) of the PPACA, which directs the Secretary to develop guidelines to provide for a de minimis variance in the actuarial valuations used in determining the level of coverage of a plan to account for differences in actuarial estimates, and section 1321(a)(1)(A) and (D) of the PPACA, which requires the Secretary to issue regulations setting standards for meeting the requirements for the establishment and operation of Exchanges, as well as such other requirements as the Secretary determines appropriate, we are finalizing the definition of the AV de minimis range included in §156.140(c) to be a variation of ¥4/+2 percentage points for all non-grandfathered individual and small group market insurance plans (other than bronze plans meeting certain conditions) that are required to comply with AV, starting with plan years beginning in 2018. Because of the urgent need to stabilize the market and attract and retain issuers to ensure that consumers have options for coverage in the 2018 Exchanges, we do not believe that consulting stakeholders in advance of finalizing the rule is necessary at this time, but we hope to engage stakeholders on what, if any, modifications are needed to publicly available data as a result of this change.

Furthermore, we are also finalizing the de minimis range change for bronze plans that either cover and pay for at least one major service, other than preventive services, before the deductible or meet the requirements to be a high deductible health plan within the meaning of 26 U.S.C. 223(c)(2) from ¥2/+5 percentage points to ¥4/+5 percentage points to align with the policy in this rule, starting in plan year 2018. We recognize that the difference between the bronze and silver plans under this de minimis range is only 1 percent and that AVs typically increase each year; therefore, we may consider further changes to the de minimis ranges in the future as we intend to monitor the effects in 2018. We also recognize that States are the enforcers of AV policy and nothing under this policy precludes States from applying stricter standards, consistent with Federal law. For example, a State may apply a +/¥2 percent for the AV de minimis range for metal level plans, which would be tied to the metal level definitions under section 1302(d)(1) of the PPACA, would be within the Federal de minimis range, and would be considered a stricter standard than the Federal requirements. However, a State cannot require issuers to design plans that apply an AV range that is not consistent with our implementation of section 1302(d)(1) and (d)(3) of the PPACA (which defines the metal level definitions). Also, it is the responsibility of the State to enforce implementation of a de minimis range using the Federal AV Calculator or an AV Calculator that utilizes State-specific data under §156.135(e).[59]

Comment: Many commenters were opposed to the proposed policy or were concerned about the potential impact on increasing cost sharing for consumers, especially in the form of higher deductibles, an area where commenters noted consumers, are already struggling. These commenters were also concerned about potential decreases in the amount of APTCs[60] that most Exchange consumers use to purchase coverage, particularly for those consumers between 250 and 400 percent of FPL who are not eligible for the current CSR silver plan variations. Many commenters generally believed that the proposed policy would reduce the value of coverage by making it less affordable; for example, a decrease in APTC could affect current enrollees' ability to stay in their current plan without having to pay more in premiums, or could affect consumers' use of services due to higher cost sharing and the associated financial implications. Some commenters commented on the lack of value of coverage for enrollees who do not receive APTCs given the high cost of coverage. Some commenters stated that a silver plan is defined in the statute as a plan with a 70 percent AV plan and supported requiring that the second lowest cost silver plan (the benchmark plan), which is used to calculate

APTCs, have an AV of at least 70 percent. Some commenters recommended finalizing a de minimis range that ensures that a change in de minimis range does not impact AV for silver plans that are used to calculate the benchmark plan for PTCs, or recommended increasing the de minimis range on only bronze plans. Other commenters noted that the proposed policy would not affect bronze plans due to the annual limitation on cost sharing, limiting the ability of a bronze plan to have a lower AV. Some commenters supported a silver plan variation eligible for CSRs at the 70 percent AV level, with some commenters believing that a 66 percent AV does not meet the statutory requirements at section 1402 of the PPACA, with some recommending that HHS establish a 70 percent plan or ensure that plans with a 70 percent AV are available, and some commenters wanted further details on the proposal to establish a 70 percent AV silver plan variation. Other commenters did not support requiring an additional silver plan variation eligible for CSRs at the 70 percent AV level due to administrative and cost burden to issuers and the absence of regulations that support an additional silver variation, and also because the reasoning in the 2012 Bulletin still applies, given that the reduction in the out-of-pocket limit would cause increases in other cost sharing. Some commented on the policy's impact on enrollees in CSR plans and on enrollees in zero cost share plans that typically use APTCs to enroll in bronze plans.

Response: In response to comments, we considered limiting this policy to the bronze level of coverage or excluding the silver level of coverage to ensure that this policy does not affect APTCs. However, we believe that limiting the policy in either way would significantly blunt the impact of the policy. As discussed in the preamble of the proposed 2018 Payment Notice, all plans subject to the annual limitation on cost sharing under section 1302(c) of the PPACA have a minimum level of generosity that limits the lowest AV that a plan can achieve, which means that issuers would not receive much additional flexibility if the expanded de minimis range were only applied to bronze plans. Because of the annual limitation on cost sharing, issuers have limited ability to design a bronze plan with an AV lower than 58.54 percent.[61] Therefore, we believe that if this policy was limited to bronze plans, the policy would likely not affect the market. Also, if the policy did not apply to silver plans, the policy would have limited impact because it would only provide issuers with significant flexibility for plans with gold and platinum levels of coverage.

Based on the Exchange plan and enrollment numbers from 2016 and 2017, there are significantly more plans and more enrollees in the silver and bronze tiers than in the gold and platinum tiers. Additionally, we do not believe that gold and platinum plans are the levels of coverage most likely to attract healthy enrollees to enter the risk pool.

In finalizing the ¥4/+2 percent for the de minimis range for all metal levels (other than bronze plans meeting certain conditions), we recognize that, in the short run, this change would generate a transfer of costs from consumers to issuers, but believe the additional flexibility for issuers will have positive effects for consumers over the longer term. Similar to the ¥2 percent de minimis range flexibility that we have previously provided for AV, the change to allow for ¥4 percent de minimis range could reduce the value of coverage for consumers compared to a narrower de minimis range, which could lead to more consumers facing increases in out-of-pocket expenses, thus increasing their exposure to financial risks associated with high medical costs. However, providing issuers with additional flexibility could help stabilize premiums over time, increase issuer participation, and ultimately provide consumers with more coverage options at the silver level and above, thereby attracting more young and healthy enrollees into plans at these levels.

In the short term, the benchmark plans used to calculate the amount of APTCs available to consumers below 400 percent of FPL could be based on a plan at the lower end of the new de minimis range that has lower premiums, meaning that a lower APTC amount could be available to all consumers eligible for APTC to retain current coverage. The impact of the policy is dependent on which plans consumers choose to enroll in and the plans that are available in the market. Consumers whose APTC decreases could instead choose a plan with lower premiums to mitigate an increase in the amount of premium they owe, but that plan may have higher cost sharing to offset the decrease in premium. Specifically, enrollees who choose to use their APTC amounts to purchase coverage for lower priced plans, such as bronze or lowest cost silver, could also be negatively impacted. Assuming issuers offer silver metal tier plans at the lower end of the new de minimis range, when individuals who are eligible for CSRs choose the silver plan variations, there could be an increase of CSRs for the lower AV plan to reach the plan variation's AV. Individuals with a household income up to 250 percent of FPL, who enroll in a CSR silver plan variation, will receive additional CSRs to make up the difference between the lower AV of the standard silver plan and the CSR silver plan variation. Individuals with a household income in the range of 250 to 400 percent of FPL do not currently receive CSRs and cannot choose to enroll in a silver plan variation will experience greater out of pocket expenses. Previously, providing a reduced maximum annual limitation on cost sharing for a 70 percent AV plan would have resulted in an AV of the standard silver plan being outside of the de minimis range unless substantive increases to other cost-sharing parameters are made. These individuals in the range of 250 to 400 percent of FPL may be affected by the policy finalized in this rule because they will not have the choice to enroll in CSR silver plan variations to cover the difference from the increased cost sharing from the standard silver plan.

As discussed in the proposed rule, we considered creating a new 70 percent silver plan variation for enrollees between 250 and 400 percent of FPL. In response to comments, we analyzed the effect of reducing the maximum annual limitation on cost sharing based on how we calculated the 2018 reduced maximum annual limitation on cost sharing. We found that it is possible to design plans at 66 percent AV and still be below 70 percent AV when the maximum annual limitation on cost sharing is reduced. However, we are not certain what the AV spread of plan designs will be under the finalized policy, whether issuers will in fact reduce the AVs of their base silver plans to the lower end of the de minimis range, and whether issuers will retain plan designs above the 70 percent AV range. Therefore, we intend to monitor 2018 standard silver plan designs to consider whether to require a 70 percent silver plan variation or explore other potential means of mitigating the effect on affordability for enrollees. For this reason, we are not changing the CSR silver plan variation policy for enrollees with incomes between 250 to 400 percent of FPL or coordinating with IRS to change the way the benchmark plans are determined for 2018, but we may explore whether we can do so in the future.

Comment: Some commenters supported the policy for 2018, and some commenters did not support applying the policy in 2018. Some commenters noted concerns about 2018 State filing deadlines. Some commenters requested a revised AV Calculator as soon as possible, and some commenters noted that the policy could help plans affected by the AV Calculator changes.

Response: As discussed in the proposed rule, we believe that changing the AV de minimis range will help retain and attract issuers to the non-grandfathered individual and small group markets, which will increase competition and choice for consumers, and therefore believe it is important to finalize the change for 2018. We agree with commenters that increased flexibility in the de minimis range could be helpful for plans affected by AV Calculator changes. Furthermore, while we recognize that AVs typically increase each year, flexibility in the de minimis range will give these plans greater flexibility to grow in future years. We appreciate the importance of releasing a revised AV Calculator, and are releasing the revised AV Calculator concurrently with this rule.[62] Because the AV range is widening and not narrowing, we believe that the policy will not create difficulties in meeting the State filing deadlines.

Comment: Some commenters commented on the potential impact of the proposed policy on plan competition, on whether the proposed policy would increase or decrease enrollment or premiums including among consumers that may receive a decreased APTC amount, or on whether the issuer or the consumer would ultimately benefit under the proposed policy with some commenters raising concerns about the purpose and impact of the policy discussed in the proposed rule. Some commenters questioned the impact of the proposed policy on risk adjustment and on current plans being considered the same plan. Other commenters commented on applying a de minimis range similar to the proposed policy to dental plans, and others submitted comments beyond the scope of the proposed rule.

Response: The risk adjustment model uses metal level specific simulated plan liability to predict estimated plan expenditures. The model plan designs used to derive plan liability are based on representative plans offered by issuers in each metal tier. Given that the risk adjustment model estimates relative differences in plan liability to calculate risk adjustment transfers and payments based on plan risk that may not have been incorporated in rate setting, we believe the risk adjustment methodology will continue to function as intended to compensate issuers based on relative differences in health risk of enrollees. However, in instances where the AV gap between two metal tiers is smaller than previously allowed, it is possible that the simulated plan liability expenditure differences between metal tiers may not be representative of plans offered.

Additionally, although issuers may offer plans at the lower end of the updated de minimis range to obtain competitive advantage, because the risk adjustment transfer formula is based on relative plan level differences, and incorporates metal level AV, it will continue to preserve the calculation of transfers based on relative differences in health risk of enrollees across plans. Similarly, the induced utilization factors in the current risk adjustment transfer formula represent relative differences between the plans and we do not believe the relative differences will be affected by the changes in the de minimis range. Therefore, we are not making any changes to the risk adjustment methodology to accommodate the changes to the de minimis range at this time. We intend to monitor the impact of asymmetric changes to the de minimis range on plan benefit designs offered, and any impacts on risk adjustment methodology and transfer formula calculations. Additionally, as we have noted in the 2018 Payment Notice, we anticipate reexamining the induced utilization factors in the future as the enrollee-level data from the risk adjustment program becomes available.

Under the exceptions to guaranteed renewability for uniform modification of coverage under §147.106(e), an issuer may, only at the time of coverage renewal, modify the health insurance coverage for a product offered in the individual market or small group market if the modification is consistent with State law and is effective uniformly for all individuals or group health plans with that product. To be considered a uniform modification of coverage, among other things, each plan within the product that has been modified must have the same cost-sharing structure as before the modification, except any variation in cost sharing solely related to changes in cost and utilization of medical care, or to maintain the same metal tier level described in sections 1302(d) and (e) of the PPACA. States have flexibility to broaden what cost- sharing changes are considered within the scope of a uniform modification of coverage and may, for example, consider uniform cost-sharing changes that result in plans having the same metal level based on the expanded de minimis range to be uniform modifications.

We intend to monitor the impact of this policy on plan design and by extension, Exchange enrollment to consider whether further changes are needed. We may also consider similar changes for dental plans in the future.

2. Network Adequacy (§156.230)

In recognition of the traditional role States have in developing and enforcing network adequacy standards, we proposed to rely on State reviews for network adequacy in States in which an FFE is operating, provided the State has a sufficient network adequacy review process. For the 2018 plan year, we proposed to defer to the States' reviews in States with the authority that is at least equal to the "reasonable access standard" identified in §156.230 and means to assess issuer network adequacy.

We also proposed a change to our approach to reviewing network adequacy in States that do not have the authority and means to conduct sufficient network adequacy reviews. In those States, we would, for the 2018 plan year, apply a standard similar to the one used in the 2014 plan year.[63] As HHS did in 2014, in States without the authority or means to conduct sufficient network adequacy reviews, we proposed for 2018 to rely on an issuer's accreditation (commercial, Medicaid, or Exchange) from an HHS-recognized accrediting entity. HHS has previously recognized three accrediting entities for the accreditation of QHPs: The National Committee for Quality Assurance, URAC, and Accreditation Association for Ambulatory Health Care.[64][65] We proposed to utilize these same three accrediting entities for network adequacy reviews for the 2018 plan year. Unaccredited issuers would be required to submit an access plan as part of the QHP Application. To show that the QHP's network meets the requirement in §156.230(a)(2), the access plan would need to demonstrate that an issuer has standards and procedures in place to maintain an adequate network consistent with the National Association of Insurance Commissioners' (NAIC's) Health Benefit Plan Network Access and Adequacy Model Act.[66]

We proposed that we would further coordinate with States to monitor network adequacy, for example, through complaint tracking. We also noted that we intended to release an updated timeline for the QHP certification process for plan year 2018 that would provide issuers with additional time to implement changes that are finalized prior to the 2018 coverage year. This new timeline was released on February 17, 2017,[67] with a version that includes finalized dates for rate review being released concurrently with this rule.

We are finalizing the changes as proposed. The following is a summary of the public comments received on the network adequacy proposed provisions and our responses:

Comment: Many commenters supported the proposal to rely on States with a sufficient network adequacy review process, to rely on an issuer's accreditation in States without a sufficient network adequacy review process, and the submission of access plans in States without sufficient review for issuers that are unaccredited. Many commenters also supported HHS no longer employing the time and distance standard. Some commenters recommended that all compliance and complaint tracking should be handled solely by States to avoid duplicative oversight and stated that States are better positioned to monitor networks.

Response: We appreciate commenters' support of our proposed policy and are finalizing the proposals as proposed. We believe this approach affirms the traditional role of States in overseeing network adequacy standards.

Comment: One commenter recommended that HHS rely on State review of network adequacy for SADPs in all States, rather than applying an accreditation standard to SADPs in States that do not have network adequacy review authority, because dental issuers do not get accredited.

Response: In States that are determined to not have sufficient network adequacy review, HHS will require SADPs to submit an access plan that demonstrates that the issuer has standards and procedures in place to maintain an adequate network consistent with NAIC's Health Benefit Plan Network Access and Adequacy Model Act (NAIC Model Act).

Comment: Many other commenters opposed the proposed change to rely primarily on State review of network adequacy and raised concerns that this could decrease healthcare access and create disparities in access to and quality of providers for consumers depending on their State or could lead to narrow networks.

Response: We appreciate the concerns, and recognize the importance of patients having access to adequate networks. However, we believe that States are best positioned to determine what constitutes an adequate network in their geographic area. We do not believe relying on State reviews in States that have the authority and means to conduct sufficient network adequacy reviews will translate to decreased access to providers. We look forward to working closely with States in this area as we implement the new network adequacy review approach. We also plan to continue to monitor the States' implementation of the NAIC Model Act, and we intend to use that information to shape future network adequacy policy. We also plan to provide information to issuers about which States have been determined not to have sufficient network adequacy processes in the near future.

Comment: Some commenters stated that accreditation is not a substitute for a robust provider network and that accreditation organizations can only revoke accreditation and do not provide ongoing oversight of QHP issuers and advocated for the continuation of time and distance criteria. One State commented that it relies on HHS for the evaluation of network adequacy and questioned if relying upon the issuer's accreditation will be sufficient.

Response: We appreciate the comments regarding these concerns. Accredited issuers are required to develop reasonable standards for access and availability of services and measure themselves against those standards. Further, we believe that the requirement for unaccredited issuers to submit an access plan to demonstrate that an issuer has standards and procedures in place to maintain an adequate network consistent with the NAIC Model Act will ensure an issuer has a sufficient provider network. We are finalizing this proposal as proposed.

3. Essential Community Providers (§156.235)

Essential community providers (ECPs) include providers that serve predominantly low-income and medically underserved individuals, and specifically include providers described in section 340B of the PHS Act and section 1927(c)(1)(D)(i)(IV) of the Act. Section 156.235 establishes requirements for inclusion of ECPs in QHP provider networks and provides an alternate standard for issuers that provide a majority of covered services through employed physicians or a single contracted medical group.

For conducting upcoming reviews of the ECP standard for QHP and SADP certification for the 2018 plan year, we proposed to follow the approach 68previously finalized in the 2018 Payment Notice and outlined in the 2018 Letter to Issuers in the Federally- facilitated Marketplaces, with two changes as outlined below. States performing plan management functions in the FFEs would be permitted to use a similar approach.

Section 156.235(a)(2)(i) stipulates that a plan has a sufficient number and geographic distribution of ECPs if it demonstrates, among other criteria, that the network includes as participating practitioners at least a minimum percentage, as specified by HHS. For the 2014 plan year, we set this minimum percentage at 20 percent, but, starting with the 2015 Letter to Issuers in the Federally-facilitated Marketplaces, we increased the minimum percentage to 30 percent.[34] For certification for the 2018 plan year, we proposed to return to the percentage used in the 2014 plan year, and to again consider the issuer to have satisfied the regulatory standard if the issuer contracts with at least 20 percent of available ECPs in each plan's service area to participate in the plan's provider network. The calculation methodology outlined in the 2018 Letter to Issuers in the Federally-facilitated Marketplaces and 2018 Payment Notice would remain unchanged.

We stated that we believe this standard will substantially reduce the regulatory burden on issuers while preserving adequate access to care provided by ECPs. In particular, as noted in the proposed rule, the standard would result in fewer issuers needing to submit a justification to prove that they include in their provider networks a sufficient number and geographic distribution of ECPs to meet the standard in §156.235. For the 2017 plan year, 6 percent of issuers were required to submit such a justification. Although none of their networks met the 30 percent ECP threshold, all of these justifications were deemed sufficient, and each network would have met the 20 percent threshold. We anticipate that issuers will readily be able to contract with at least 20 percent of ECPs in a service area, and that enrollees will have reasonable and timely access to ECPs.

For certification for the 2018 plan year, we also proposed to modify our previous guidance regarding which providers issuers may identify as ECPs within their provider networks. Under our current guidance, issuers would only be able to identify providers in their network who are included on a list of available ECPs maintained by HHS ("the HHS ECP list"). This list is based on data maintained by HHS, including provider data that HHS receives directly from providers through the ECP petition process for the 2018 plan year.[69] In previous years, we also permitted issuers to identify ECPs through a write- in process. Because the ECP petition process is intended to ensure qualified ECPs are included in the HHS ECP list, we indicated in guidance that we would not allow issuers to submit ECP write-ins for plan year 2018. However, we are aware that not all qualified ECPs have submitted an ECP petition, and therefore have determined the write-in process is still needed to allow issuers to identify all ECPs in their network. Therefore, as for plan year 2017, for plan year 2018, we proposed that an issuer's ECP write-ins would count toward the satisfaction of the ECP standard only for the issuer that wrote in the ECP on its ECP template, provided that the issuer arranges that the written-in provider has submitted an ECP petition to HHS by no later than the deadline for issuer submission of changes to the QHP application. For example, issuers may write in any providers that are currently eligible to participate in the 340B Drug Program described in section 340B of the PHS Act[70] that are not included on the HHS list, or not-for-profit or State-owned providers that would be entities described in section 340B of the PHS Act but do not receive Federal funding under the relevant section of law referred to in section 340B of the PHS Act, as long as the provider has submitted a timely ECP petition. Such providers include not-for-profit or governmental family planning service sites that do not receive a grant under Title X of the PHS Act. We believe the proposal would help build the HHS ECP list so that it is more inclusive of qualified ECPs and better recognize issuers for the ECPs with whom they contract.

As in previous years, if an issuer's application does not satisfy the ECP standard, the issuer would be required to include as part of its application for QHP certification a satisfactory narrative justification describing how the issuer's provider networks, as presently constituted, provide an adequate level of service for low-income and medically underserved individuals and how the issuer plans to increase ECP participation in the issuer's provider networks in future years. At a minimum, such narrative justification would include the number of contracts offered to ECPs for the 2018 plan year; the number of additional contracts an issuer expects to offer and the timeframe of those planned negotiations; the names of the specific ECPs to which the issuer has offered contracts that are still pending; and contingency plans for how the issuer's provider network, as currently designed, would provide adequate care to enrollees who might otherwise be cared for by relevant ECP types that are missing from the issuer's provider network.

For the 2018 plan year, we are finalizing our proposals to decrease the minimum ECP threshold from 30 to 20 percent of the available ECPs in a plan's service area, and to continue to allow an issuer's ECP write-ins to count toward the satisfaction of the ECP standard for only the issuer that wrote in the ECP on its ECP template, provided that the issuer arranges that the written-in provider has submitted an ECP petition to HHS by no later than the deadline for issuer submission of changes to the QHP application.

Comment: Several commenters supported our proposal to decrease the minimum ECP threshold from 30 to 20 percent, stating that the lower threshold requirement would reduce the administrative burden on issuers, especially for those issuers in rural areas or States with few ECPs.

Other commenters recommended that HHS further lower the ECP threshold to 15 percent for dental issuers, due to fewer ECPs that offer dental services.

Response: We appreciate these comments and agree that the lower 20 percent threshold requirement would reduce the administrative burden on issuers without affecting the ability of low-income and medically-underserved individuals to receive reasonable and timely access to care. At this time, we do not believe lowering the ECP threshold to 15 percent for dental issuers would adequately promote patient access to dental ECPs, given that there are fewer available dental ECPs compared to medical ECPs for low- income and medically-underserved consumers to access dental care.

Comment: Many commenters opposed our proposal to decrease the minimum ECP threshold that an issuer must achieve from 30 to 20 percent of the number of available ECPs located in a plan's service area. These commenters expressed concerns that the lower threshold requirement would result in access barriers to care for low-income consumers; restricted access to specialty care; dangerous and costly treatment interruptions; continuity of care challenges; increased travel time; poor access to culturally appropriate healthcare providers; and diminished access to community health centers, safety net and children's hospitals, HIV/ AIDS clinics, and family planning health centers. Many of these commenters stated that lowering the ECP threshold to achieve a reduced administrative burden on issuers is unnecessary given that 94 percent of issuers satisfied the 30 percent threshold for plan year 2017 and the remaining 6 percent were able to submit a satisfactory justification to meet the ECP regulatory requirement. Several commenters opposed the reduction in the threshold requirement, stating that the 30 percent threshold for plan year 2017 was not high enough to provide sufficient access to ECPs. One commenter supported the decrease of the ECP threshold for States with issuers that experienced difficulty satisfying the 30 percent threshold, but suggested that States with issuers that did not experience any difficulty be given the flexibility to require a higher ECP percent threshold.

Response: We are finalizing our proposal to decrease the ECP threshold requirement from 30 to 20 percent for plan year 2018 in an effort to reduce the regulatory burden on issuers and stabilize the Exchanges. The final rule provides that this threshold will be applicable for the 2018 plan year. Given the recent refinements to the HHS ECP list through the ECP petition process (for example, the addition of newly qualified ECPs and the removal of former ECPs that no longer provide care to low-income, medically-underserved populations), a 20 percent ECP threshold requirement is expected to adequately protect consumer access to ECPs for plan year 2018, while reducing the issuer burden that was associated with heavier reliance on the ECP write- in process to achieve the 94 percent issuer compliance with the 30 percent threshold for plan year 2017. We appreciate the suggestion to provide States with issuers that did not experience any difficulty achieving the 30 percent threshold the flexibility to require a higher ECP percent threshold. However, because the lower threshold reduces issuer burden while adequately protecting consumer access to ECPs, we believe it is important that this change apply in all States with FFEs.

Comment: All commenters supported the proposal to continue the ECP write- in process for the 2018 plan year using the ECP petition process. Some commenters stated that it would reduce administrative burden by continuing to allow issuers to count providers they have contracted with for the 2018 plan year but who missed the ECP petition window for the final 2018 plan year ECP list. Other commenters appreciated the additional time for providers to petition to be added to the HHS ECP list. Several commenters urged that we sunset the ECP write-in process for the 2019 plan year and beyond, allowing the 2018 plan year to further refine the ECP petition process.

Response: We are finalizing our proposal to continue the ECP write-in process for the 2018 plan year using the ECP petition process. We agree with commenters that continuation of the ECP write-in process for the 2018 plan year using the ECP petition process will ensure that issuers are better recognized for the ECPs with whom they contract by offering those providers additional time to petition for inclusion on the HHS ECP list. We appreciate commenters' recommendations regarding the appropriate time to sunset the ECP write-in process, and will take these into consideration in the future.

Comment: Numerous commenters urged that HHS extend the continuity of care protections under §156.230(d) to ECP discontinuations from the issuer's provider network across plan years. These commenters stated that extending continuity of care provisions to ECPs would have negligible impact on issuers because issuers must already follow these requirements for provider discontinuations within a plan year.

Commenters further explained that this protection would discourage discriminatory benefit design and support enrollee continuance within the same plan, promoting market stability. Without these protections, commenters expressed concern that issuers will attempt to shed high-cost enrollees by eliminating their ECPs from the provider network.

Response: In the 2017 Payment Notice (81 FR 12204), we finalized two policies related to continuity of care at §156.230(d), which began applying in 2017 and apply to ECP terminations. First, we require the issuer, under §156.230(d)(1), to make a good faith effort to provide written notice of discontinuation of a provider 30 days prior to the effective date of the change, or otherwise as soon as practicable, to enrollees who are patients seen on a regular basis by the provider or who receive primary care from the provider whose contract is being discontinued, irrespective of whether the contract is being discontinued due to a termination for cause or without cause, or due to a nonrenewal. Second, in cases where a provider is terminated without cause, we require the issuer, under §156.230(d)(2), to allow enrollees in an active course of treatment to continue treatment until the treatment is complete or for 90 days, whichever is shorter, at in-network cost-sharing rates. These policies apply to provider transitions that occur because a QHP issuer in an FFE discontinues its contract with an ECP. More explicitly, with respect to §156.230(d)(1), this policy applies to ECP contract discontinuations, irrespective of whether the contract is being discontinued due to a termination for cause or without cause, or due to a non- renewal; and with respect to §156.230(d)(2), this policy applies to ECP contract discontinuations where a provider is terminated without cause. **IV.**

Provisions of the Final Regulations

For the most part, this final rule incorporates the provisions of the proposed rule. However, this final rule makes clarifications to the scope of the guaranteed availability policy regarding unpaid premiums; makes modifications to the provisions relating to special enrollment periods; finalizes amendments to §155.400 to conform to changes made in this rule; and makes clarifications regarding States' roles.

V. Collection of Information Requirements

Under the Paperwork Reduction Act of 1995, we are required to provide 30- day notice in the **Federal Register** and solicit public comment before a collection of information requirement is submitted to the Office of Management and Budget (OMB) for review and approval. This final rule contains information collection requirements (ICRs) that are subject to review by OMB. A description of these provisions is given in the following paragraphs, with an estimate of the annual burden. To fairly evaluate whether an information collection should be approved by OMB, section 3506(c)(2)(A) of the Paperwork Reduction Act of 1995 requires that we solicit comments on the following issues:

- The need for the information collection and its usefulness in carrying out the proper functions of our agency.
- The accuracy of our estimate of the information collection burden.
- The quality, utility, and clarity of the information to be collected.
- Recommendations to minimize the information collection burden on the affected public, including automated collection techniques.

We solicited public comment on each of these issues for the following sections of the proposed rule that contain ICRs.

A. ICRs Regarding Verification of Eligibility for Special Enrollment Periods (§155.420)

Starting in June 2017, HHS will begin to implement pre-enrollment verification of eligibility for all categories of special enrollment periods for all States served by the *HealthCare.gov* platform. Currently, individuals self-attest to their eligibility for many special enrollment periods and submit supporting documentation, but enroll in coverage through the Exchanges without any pre-enrollment verification. As mentioned in the preamble to this rule, beginning in June 2017, we previously planned to implement a pilot program to conduct pre-enrollment verification for a sample of 50 percent of consumers attempting to enroll in coverage through special enrollment periods. We will now expand pre-enrollment verification to all new consumers for applicable special enrollment periods, so that enrollment will be delayed or "pended" until verification of eligibility is completed. Individuals will have to provide supporting documentation within 30 days. Where possible, the FFE will make every effort to verify an individual's eligibility for the applicable special enrollment period through automated electronic means instead of through a consumer's submission of documentation. Since consumers currently provide required supporting documentation even though there is no pre-enrollment verification process, the provisions will not impose any additional paperwork burden on consumers.

Based on enrollment data, we estimate that HHS eligibility support staff members will conduct pre- enrollment verification for an additional 650,000 individuals. Once individuals have submitted the required verification documents, we estimate that it will take approximately 12 minutes (at an hourly cost of $40.82) to review and verify submitted verification documents. The verification process will result in an additional annual burden for the Federal government of 130,000 hours at a cost of $5,306,600.

We have revised the information collection currently approved under OMB control number 0938–1207 (Medicaid and Children's Health Insurance Programs: Essential Health Benefits in Alternative Benefit Plans,

Eligibility Notices, Fair Hearing and Appeal Processes, and Premiums and Cost Sharing; Exchanges: Eligibility and Enrollment) to account for this additional burden. The 30-day notice soliciting public comment will be published in the **Federal Register** at a future date.

SBEs that currently do not conduct pre-enrollment verification for special enrollment periods are encouraged to follow the same approach. States that choose to do so will change their current approach. Under 5 CFR 1320.3(c)(4), this ICR is not subject to the PRA as we anticipate it would affect fewer than 10 entities in a 12-month period.

Comment: Commenters expressed concerns about the lack of Federal staff and resources available to adjudicate documents in a timely manner, especially when the work is layered on top of ongoing post-enrollment documentation verification for inconsistencies. Commenters noted the increased costs to the Federal government due to increased staffing needs and secure storage of submitted documents, and the additional time both consumers and assisters will need to spend to adhere to these new requirements. A few commenters indicated that a pre-enrollment verification of special enrollment period eligibility may also affect other entities, such as issuers and medical providers who would incur costs in re-submitting or refiling claims, processing retroactive claims, and effectuating retroactive enrollments. One commenter suggested that

HHS's cost analysis include these costs, as well as the consumer cost of spending time requesting that claims be re-billed.

Response: We appreciate the concerns about the increased burden and cost that a documentation requirement for pre- enrollment verification of eligibility for special enrollment periods will have on all entities involved. We are dedicated to reviewing all special enrollment period documents received as quickly as possible in order to minimize delays. Although we recognize that gathering and submitting these documents can be difficult and time consuming, we do not believe that this places a new burden on consumers or those providing enrollment assistance since consumers are already required to submit documentation to prove their eligibility after enrollment for 5 common special enrollment periods. Because of our plans for timely document review, we do not believe that new costs will be incurred by issuers, medical providers, or consumers needing to re-submit, refile, or re-bill for claims for services received due to this new requirement.

B. ICRs Regarding Network Adequacy Reviews and Essential Community Providers (§156.230, §156.235)

After further review and consideration, HHS has determined that the ICRs associated with QHP certification have already been assessed and encompassed by CMS-10592/OMB Control No. 0938-1187 (Establishment of Exchanges and Qualified Health Plans; Exchange Standards for Employers). As such, the proposed ICRs related to QHP certification in the proposed rule have been removed in this final rule.

VI. Regulatory Impact Analysis

A. Statement of Need

As noted previously in the preamble, the Exchanges have experienced a decrease in the number of participating issuers and many States have recently seen increases in premiums. This final rule, which is being published as issuers develop their proposed plan benefit structures and premiums for 2018, aims to improve market stability and issuer participation in the Exchanges for the 2018 benefit year and beyond. This rule also aims to reduce the fiscal and regulatory burden on individuals, families, health insurers, patients, recipients of healthcare services, and purchasers of health insurance. This rule seeks to lower insurance rates and ensure dynamic and competitive markets in part by preventing and curbing potential misuse and abuse associated with special enrollment periods and gaming by individuals taking advantage of the current regulations on grace periods and termination of coverage due to the non-payment of premiums.

This rule addresses these issues by changing a number of requirements that HHS believes will provide needed flexibility to issuers and help stabilize the individual insurance markets, allowing consumers in many State or local markets to retain or obtain health insurance while incentivizing issuers to enter, or remain, in these markets while returning greater autonomy to the States for a number of issues.

B.   Overall Impact

We have examined the impacts of this rule as required by Executive Order 12866 on Regulatory Planning and Review (September 30, 1993), Executive Order 13563 on Improving Regulation and Regulatory Review (January 18, 2011), the Regulatory Flexibility Act (RFA) (September 19, 1980, Pub. L. 96- 354), section 202 of the Unfunded Mandates Reform Act of 1995 (March 22, 1995, Pub. L. 104-4), Executive Order 13132 on Federalism (August 4, 1999), the Congressional Review Act (5 U.S.C. 804(2)), and Executive Order 13771 on Reducing Regulation and Controlling Regulatory Costs (January 30, 2017). Executive Orders 12866 and 13563 direct agencies to assess all costs and benefits of available regulatory alternatives and, if regulation is necessary, to select regulatory approaches that maximize net benefits (including potential economic, environmental, public health and safety effects, distributive impacts, and equity). Executive Order 13563 emphasizes the importance of quantifying both costs and benefits, of reducing costs, of harmonizing rules, and of promoting flexibility.

Section 3(f) of Executive Order 12866 defines a "significant regulatory action" as an action that is likely to result in a rule — (1) having an annual effect on the economy of $100 million or more in any 1 year, or adversely and materially affecting a sector of the economy, productivity, competition, jobs, the environment, public health or safety, or State, local or tribal governments or communities (also referred to as "economically significant"); (2) creating a serious inconsistency or otherwise interfering with an action taken or planned by another agency; (3) materially altering the budgetary impacts of entitlement grants, user fees, or loan programs or the rights and obligations of recipients thereof; or (4) raising novel legal or policy issues arising out of legal mandates, the President's priorities, or the principles set forth in the Executive Order.

A regulatory impact analysis (RIA) must be prepared for major rules with economically significant effects ($100 million or more in any 1 year), and a "significant" regulatory action is subject to review by OMB. HHS has concluded that this rule is likely to have economic impacts of $100 million or more in at least 1 year, and therefore, meets the definition of "significant rule" under Executive Order 12866. Therefore, HHS has provided an assessment of the potential costs, benefits, and transfers associated with this rule.

The provisions in this final rule aim to improve the health and stability of the Exchanges. They provide additional flexibility to issuers for plan designs, reduce regulatory burden, reduce administrative costs, seek to improve issuer risk pools and lower premiums by reducing potential gaming and adverse selection and incentivize consumers to maintain continuous coverage. Through the reduction in financial uncertainty for issuers and increased affordability for consumers, these provisions are expected to increase access to affordable health coverage. Although there is some uncertainty regarding the net effect on enrollment, premiums, and total premium tax credit payments by the government, we anticipate that the provisions of this final rule will help further HHS's goal of ensuring that all consumers have quality, affordable healthcare; that markets are stable; and that Exchanges operate smoothly.

In accordance with Executive Order 12866, HHS has determined that the benefits of this regulatory action justify the costs.

C. Impact Estimates and Accounting Table

In accordance with OMB Circular A-4, Table 1 depicts an accounting statement summarizing HHS's assessment of the benefits, costs, and transfers associated with this regulatory action.

The provisions in this rule will have a number of effects, including reducing regulatory burden for issuers, reducing the impact of adverse selection, stabilizing premiums in the individual insurance markets, and providing consumers with more affordable health insurance coverage. The effects in Table 1 reflect qualitative impacts and estimated direct monetary costs and transfers resulting from the provisions of this final rule.

Benefits:

Qualitative:
- Improved health and protection from the risk of catastrophic medical expenditures for the previously uninsured, especially individuals with medical conditions (if health insurance enrollment increases).[a]
- Cost savings due to reduction in providing medical services (if health insurance enrollment decreases).[ab]
- Cost savings to issuers from not having to process claims while enrollment is "pended" during pre-enrollment verification of eligibility for special enrollment periods.[c]
- Cost savings to the government and plans associated with the reduced open enrollment period.
- Costs savings to consumers and issuers due reduced administrative costs to issuers.

Costs:

Qualitative:
- Harms to health and reduced protection from the risk of catastrophic medical expenditures for the previously uninsured, especially individuals with medical conditions (if health insurance enrollment decreases).a
- Cost due to increases in providing medical services (if health insurance enrollment increases).ab
- Possible decrease in quality of medical services (for example, reductions in continuity of care due to lower ECP threshold).
- Administrative costs incurred by the Federal government and by States that start conducting verification of special enrollment period eligibility.
- Costs to issuers of redesigning plans.
- Costs to the Federal government and issuers of outreach activities associated with shortened open enrollment period.
- Administrative costs to stakeholders to read, comprehend and comply with provisions of the final rule.

Transfers	Low estimate (million)	High estimate (million)	Year dollar	Discount rate (percent)	Period covered
Annualized Monetized ($millions/year)			2016 2016	73	2018–2022 2018–2022

Transfer from Federal Government to issuers and providers via possible increases in CSRs, as well as a transfer of similar magnitude via possible reductions in APTC subsidies from some combination of enrollees and issuers to the Federal Government.

Qualitative:

- Transfers, via premium reductions and claim reductions, from special enrollment period applicants who do not provide sufficient documentation and their medical providers to all other enrollees and issuers.
- Transfers related to changes in AV from enrollees to issuers.
- Transfer from enrollees to issuers in the form of payments made for past due premiums.

Notes: [a]Enrollment may increase due to decreases in premiums resulting from pass-through of administrative cost savings (as listed) and savings associated with reductions in special enrollment period or the shortened open enrollment period. Enrollment may decrease due to lessened consumer appeal of insurance with reduced AV and less access to ECPs, increases in premiums resulting from pass-through of administrative costs (as listed), former special enrollment period users discontinuing participation, or due to shortened enrollment periods. The net effect on enrollment is ambiguous. [b]These cost and cost savings generalizations are somewhat oversimplified because uninsured individuals are relatively likely to obtain healthcare through high-cost providers (for example, visiting an emergency room for preventive services). cThese savings will potentially be negated as issuers process any claims that occur while being "pended" once an enrollee's SEP eligibility has been verified.

1. Guaranteed Availability of Coverage

This final rule provides that, to the extent permitted by applicable State law, issuers may apply a premium payment to past-due premiums owed for coverage from the same issuer, or another issuer in the same controlled group within the prior 12 month period preceding the effective date of coverage before effectuating new coverage. Individuals with past due premiums will generally owe no more than 1 to 3 months of past-due premiums. The issuer will have to apply its premium payment policy uniformly to all employers or individuals in similar circumstances in the applicable market and State and regardless of health status and consistent with applicable non- discrimination requirements. Furthermore, issuers adopting a premium payment policy, as well as any issuers that do not adopt the policy but are within an adopting issuer's controlled group, must clearly describe in any enrollment application materials and in any notice that is provided regarding non-payment of premiums, whether in paper or electronic form, the consequences of non-payment on future enrollment. Plan documents and related materials are usually reviewed and updated annually before a new plan year begins. Issuers may include this information in their plan documents and related materials at negligible cost at that time. This will reduce misuse of grace periods and the risk of adverse selection by consumers while likely also discouraging some individuals from obtaining coverage.

A recent study[37] surveying consumers with individual market plans concluded that approximately 21 percent of consumers stopped premium payments in 2015. Approximately 87 percent of those individuals repurchased plans in 2016, and 49 percent of these consumers purchased the same plan on which they had previously stopped payment.

Based on internal analysis, we estimate that approximately one in ten enrollees in the FFE had their coverage terminated due to non-payment of premiums in 2016. We estimate that approximately 86,000 (or 16 percent) of those individuals whose coverage was terminated due to non-payment of premium in 2016 and who lived in an area where their 2016 issuer was available in 2017 had an active 2017 plan selection with the same issuer at the end of the open enrollment period. Additionally, for those individuals living in an area where their 2016 issuer was the only issuer available in 2017, 23 percent of those individuals whose coverage was terminated due to non- payment in 2016 had an active 2017 plan selection with that issuer at the end of the open enrollment period— equating to approximately 21,000 individuals. In the absence of data, we are unable to determine the amount of past-due premiums that consumers will have to pay in order to effectuate new coverage with the same issuer or an issuer in the same controlled group, though individuals will generally owe no more than 1 to 3 months of premiums.

2. Open Enrollment Periods

This final rule amends §155.410(e) and changes the individual market annual open enrollment period for coverage year 2018 to begin on November 1, 2017, and run through December 15, 2017. This is expected to have a positive impact on the individual market risk pools by reducing the risk of adverse selection. However, the shortened enrollment period could lead to a reduction in enrollees, primarily younger and healthier enrollees who usually enroll late in the enrollment period. The change in the open enrollment period could lead to additional reductions in enrollment if Exchanges and enrollment assisters do not have adequate support, which can lead to potential enrollees facing longer wait times. In addition, this change is expected to simplify operational processes for issuers and the Exchanges. However, the Federal government, SBEs, and issuers may incur costs if additional consumer outreach is needed.

3. Special Enrollment Periods

Special enrollment periods ensure that people who lose health insurance during the year (for example, through non-voluntary loss of minimum essential coverage provided through an employer), or who experience other qualifying events such as marriage or birth or adoption of a child, have the opportunity to enroll in new coverage or make changes to their existing coverage. In the individual market, while the annual open enrollment period allows previously uninsured individuals to enroll in new insurance coverage, special enrollment periods are intended to promote continuous enrollment in health insurance coverage during the benefit year by allowing those who were previously enrolled in coverage to obtain new coverage without a lapse or gap in coverage.

However, allowing previously uninsured individuals to enroll in coverage via a special enrollment period that they would not otherwise qualify for can increase the risk of adverse selection, negatively impact the risk pool, contribute to gaps in coverage, and contribute to market instability and reduced issuer participation.

Currently, in many cases, individuals self-attest to their eligibility for most special enrollment periods and submit supporting documentation, but enroll in coverage through the Exchanges without further pre-enrollment verification. As mentioned earlier in the preamble, in 2016 we took several steps to further verify eligibility for special enrollment periods and planned to implement a pilot program to conduct pre-enrollment verification for a sample of 50 percent of consumers attempting to enroll in coverage through special enrollment periods. The provisions finalized in this rule will increase the scope of pre- enrollment verification, strengthen and streamline the parameters of several existing special enrollment periods, and limit several other special enrollment periods. Starting in June 2017, new consumers in all States served by the *HealthCare.gov* platform attempting to enroll through applicable special enrollment periods will have to undergo pre-enrollment verification of eligibility, so that their enrollment would be delayed or "pended" until verification of eligibility is completed by the Exchange. Where possible, the FFE will make every effort to verify an individual's eligibility for a special enrollment period through automated electronic means instead of through documentation. Based on past experience, we estimate that the expansion in pre-enrollment verification to all individuals seeking to enroll in coverage through all applicable special enrollment periods will result in an additional 650,000 individuals having their enrollment delayed or "pended" annually until eligibility verification is completed. As discussed previously in the Collection of Information Requirements section, there will be an increase in costs to the Federal government for conducting the additional pre-enrollment verifications. SBEs that begin to conduct pre-enrollment verification will incur administrative costs to conduct those reviews. We anticipate that there will be a reduction in costs to issuers since they will not have to process any claims while the enrollments are "pended", though these savings may be negated as issuers process any claims that occur while an enrollment is "pended" once an enrollee's special enrollment period eligibility has been verified.

The changes will promote continuous coverage and allow individuals who qualify for a special enrollment period to obtain coverage, while ensuring that uninsured individuals who do not qualify for a special enrollment period obtain coverage during open enrollment instead of waiting until they get sick, which is expected to protect the Exchange risk pools, enhance market stability, and in doing so, limit rate increases. On the other hand, it is possible that the additional steps required to verify eligibility may discourage some eligible individuals from obtaining coverage, and reduce access to healthcare for those individuals, increasing their exposure to financial risk. If it deters younger and healthier individuals from obtaining coverage, it can also worsen the risk pool.

If pre-enrollment verification causes premiums to fall and all individuals who inappropriately enrolled via special enrollment periods continue to be covered, there will be a transfer from such individuals to other consumers. Conversely, if some individuals are no longer able to enroll via special enrollment periods, they will experience reduced access to healthcare. If there is a significant decrease in enrollment,[71] especially for younger and healthier individuals, it is possible that premiums will not fall, and potentially might increase.

Office of the Actuary analysis of the net effect of pre-enrollment verification and other special enrollment period changes estimated that premiums will be approximately 1.5 percent lower. The premium difference was calculated by taking into account the greater claims cost per member per month for enrollees through special enrollment periods and fewer enrollees through special enrollment periods.

4. Levels of Coverage (Actuarial Value)

We are amending the de minimis range included in §156.140(c), to a variation of ¥4/+2 percentage points, rather than +/¥ 2 percentage points for all non-grandfathered individual and small group market plans (other than bronze plans meeting certain conditions) that are required to comply with AV for plans beginning in 2018. We are also amending the expanded de minimis range for certain bronze plans from ¥2/+5 percentage points to ¥4/+5 percentage points to align with the policy in this rule for the same timeline. While we are modifying the de minimis range for the metal level plans (bronze, silver, gold, and platinum), we are not modifying the de minimis range for the silver plan variations (the plans with an AV of 73, 87 and 94 percent) under §§156.400 and 156.420. In the short run, the impact of this change will be to generate a transfer of costs from consumers to issuers. The change in AV may reduce the value of coverage for consumers, which can lead to more consumers facing increases in out-of- pocket expenses, thus increasing their exposure to financial risks associated with high medical costs. However, providing issuers with additional flexibility can help stabilize premiums over time, increase issuer participation and ultimately provide more coverage options at the silver level and above, thereby attracting more young and healthy enrollees into plans at these levels.

Taking into account limits on design flexibilities for bronze plans and related to State limits on flexibility, the Office of the Actuary analysis estimated that the change in AV will lead to a 0.75 percent reduction in total premiums. This analysis estimated that the change to the de minimis range would reduce premiums for the non-subsidized population at the silver, gold, and platinum metal levels.

The lower AV will decrease plan liability for non-cost-sharing variation plans in silver, gold, and platinum and therefore premiums for non-subsidized enrollees will have a proportional reduction in premiums comparable to the reduction in AV.

A reduction in premiums will likely also reduce the benchmark premium for purposes of the premium tax credit, leading to a transfer from APTC (or premium tax credit) recipients to the government. One commenter estimated that if the AV for all benchmark silver level plans were to decrease from 68 to 66 percent AV, this would result in a decrease of the benchmark premium by $131 per year, which would reduce APTCs the Federal government provides to consumers by $381 million dollars per year (holding enrollment constant). We agree with the commenter's assessment that lower financial assistance in the form of APTCs is likely. The premium reduction measures total premium reductions not the effects of lower APTC on net premiums for subsidized enrollees. With a decrease in the benchmark premium and therefore the APTC, enrollees, particularly subsidized enrollees who purchase plans with premiums less than the second lowest cost silver plan, could have higher net premiums than in prior years.

The decrease in the de minimis range for the silver metal tier will also affect the value of cost-sharing reductions provided to individuals who qualify for CSRs, with the magnitude of the impact based on individual income levels. Currently, individuals with a household income in the range of 250 to 400 percent of FPL do not receive any CSRs because reductions to the maximum annual limitation on cost sharing under the previous de minimis range of 68 percent–72 percent AV, without substantive increases to other cost sharing parameters would have resulted in an AV that exceeded the statutory maximum 70 percent AV. Because enrollees with incomes between 250 to 400 percent of FPL do not receive CSRs, the lower AV for the silver metal tier will result in higher cost sharing for these individuals. However, individuals with a household income up to 250 percent of FPL, who enroll in a CSR silver plan variation, will benefit from additional CSRs that the issuer will provide to make up the difference between the lower AV of silver metal tier standard plans and the CSR silver plan variation AV. As part of CSR reconciliation, HHS will continue to calculate CSR amounts provided based on the cost sharing that the individual would have otherwise paid in a standard plan. That is, if the standard plan the CSR-eligible enrollee chooses is now a 66 percent AV plan, with a de minimis variation of 4 percent below 70 percent AV (or 2 percentage points below the lowest available silver plan at 68 percent AV previously), the CSRs provided will equal the difference between the value of CSRs in the applicable CSR silver plan variation (either 73 percent, 87 percent, 94 percent AV), and the standard plan (66 percent), which will be greater than the CSRs provided if the standard silver plan has +/¥2 percent allowable variation. Based on the most recent data on CSRs provided by CSR plan variations, steady-state enrollment in CSR plans, and an increase in CSRs provided based on a conservative range of 30 to 50 percent of CSR eligible individuals choosing a standard silver plan with lower AV than previously available, we estimate the lowered AV under the new de minimis range will increase the CSRs provided to enrollees in 2018 by approximately $200 million to $400 million or approximately an amount equal to the expected reduction in APTCs (or premium tax credits) described above in this section.

5. Network Adequacy

Section 156.230(a)(2) requires a QHP issuer to maintain a network that is sufficient in number and types of providers, including providers that specialize in mental health and substance abuse services, to assure that all services will be accessible without unreasonable delay. For the 2018 plan year, HHS will defer to the State's reviews in States with authority and means to assess issuer network adequacy; while in States without authority and means to conduct sufficient network adequacy reviews, HHS will rely on an issuer's accreditation (commercial, Medicaid, or Exchange) from an HHS-recognized accrediting entity. Unaccredited issuers in States without network adequacy review will be required to submit an access plan as part of the QHP Application. This may reduce administrative costs for issuers, which can ultimately lead to reduced premiums for consumers.

Depending on the level of review by State regulators and accrediting entities, this can have an impact on plan design. Issuers can potentially use network designs to encourage enrollment into certain plans, exacerbating selection pressures. The net effect on consumers is uncertain.

6. Essential Community Providers

Section 156.235(a)(2)(i) stipulates that a plan has a sufficient number and geographic distribution of ECPs if it demonstrates, among other criteria, that the network includes as participating practitioners at least a minimum percentage, as specified by HHS. For the 2014 plan year, this minimum percentage was 20 percent, but starting with the 2015 Letter to Issuers in the Federally-facilitated Marketplaces, we increased the minimum percentage to 30 percent. For certification and recertification for the 2018 plan year, we will instead consider the issuer to have satisfied the regulatory standard if the issuer contracts with at least 20 percent of available ECPs in each plan's service area to participate in the plan's provider network. In addition, we are reversing our previous guidance that we were discontinuing the write-in process for ECPs, and will continue to allow this process for the 2018 plan year. If an issuer's application does not satisfy the ECP standard, the issuer will be required to include as part of its application for QHP certification a satisfactory narrative justification describing how the issuer's provider networks, as presently constituted, provide an adequate level of service for low-income and medically underserved individuals and how the issuer plans to increase ECP participation in the issuer's provider networks in future years. We expect that issuers will be able to meet this requirement, with the exception of issuers that do not have any ECPs in their service area.

Less expansive requirements for network size will lead to both costs and cost savings. Costs can take the form of increased travel time and wait time for appointments or reductions in continuity of care for those patients whose providers have been removed from their insurance issuers' networks.

Cost savings for issuers will be associated with reductions in administrative costs of arranging contracts, meeting QHP certification requirements, and, if issuers focus their networks on relatively low-cost providers to the extent possible, reductions in the cost of healthcare provision.

7. Uncertainty

The net effect of these provisions on enrollment, premiums and total premium tax credit payments are uncertain. That is, premiums will tend to fall if more young and healthy individuals obtain coverage, adverse selection is reduced and issuers are able to lower costs due to reduced regulatory burden, and offer greater flexibility in plan design. However, if changes such as a shortened open enrollment period, pre-enrollment verification for special enrollment periods, reduced AV of plans, or less expansive provider networks result in lower enrollment, especially for younger, healthier adults, it will tend to increase premiums. Lower premiums in turn will increase enrollment, while higher premiums will have the opposite effect. In addition, lower premiums will tend to decrease total premium tax credit payments, which can be offset by an increase in enrollment. Increased enrollment will lead to an overall increase in healthcare spending by issuers, while a decrease in enrollment will lower it, although the effect on total healthcare spending is uncertain, since uninsured individuals are more likely to obtain healthcare through high cost providers such as emergency rooms.

D. *Regulatory Alternatives Considered*

In developing the final rule, we considered maintaining the status quo with respect to our interpretation of guaranteed availability, network adequacy requirements, and essential community provider requirements. However, we determined that the changes are urgently needed to stabilize markets, to incentivize issuers to enter into or remain in the market and to ensure premium stability and consumer choice.

With respect to the provision regarding essential community providers, we considered proposing a minimum threshold other than 20 percent, but believed that reverting to the previously used 20 percent threshold that issuers were used to would better help stabilize the markets, while adequately protecting access to ECPs.

We also considered keeping the current individual market open enrollment period for 2018 coverage, but determined that an immediate change would have a positive impact on the individual market risk pools by reducing the risk of adverse selection and that the market is mature enough for an immediate transition.

In addition, we considered increasing the scope of pre-enrollment verification for certain special enrollment periods to 90 percent instead of 100 percent. This would have allowed us to maximize the verification of eligibility while providing some control population for claims comparison as envisioned by the scaled pilot. We solicited comment on the issue, but noted that we believe that in order to minimize the risk of adverse selection, complete pre-enrollment verification for special enrollment periods is necessary. We also considered maintaining the existing parameters around special enrollment periods so that the individual market special enrollment periods would continue to align with group market policies. However, HHS determined that aspects of the individual market and the unique threats of adverse selection in this market justified a departure from the group market policies.

With respect to the provision regarding AV, we considered proposing that the change would be effective for the 2019 plan year, but determined that an immediate change would have a positive impact on the markets for the 2018 plan year.

E. Regulatory Flexibility Act

The Regulatory Flexibility Act (5 U.S.C. 601, *et seq.*) requires agencies to prepare a regulatory flexibility analysis to describe the impact of the proposed rule on small entities, unless the head of the agency can certify that the rule would not have a significant economic impact on a substantial number of small entities. The RFA generally defines a "small entity" as (1) a proprietary firm meeting the size standards of the Small Business Administration (SBA), (2) a not-for-profit organization that is not dominant in its field, or (3) a small government jurisdiction with a population of less than 50,000. States and individuals are not included in the definition of "small entity." HHS uses a change in revenues of more than 3 to 5 percent as its measure of significant economic impact on a substantial number of small entities.

This rule will affect health insurance issuers. We believe that health insurance issuers would be classified under the North American Industry Classification System code 524114 (Direct Health and Medical Insurance Carriers). According to SBA size standards, entities with average annual receipts of $38.5 million or less would be considered small entities for these North American Industry Classification System codes. Issuers could possibly be classified in 621491 (HMO Medical

Centers) and, if this is the case, the SBA size standard would be $32.5 million or less.[72] We believe that few, if any, insurance companies underwriting comprehensive health insurance policies (in contrast, for example, to travel insurance policies or dental discount policies) fall below these size thresholds. Based on data from MLR annual report submissions for the 2015 MLR reporting year, approximately 97 out of 528 issuers of health insurance coverage nationwide had total premium revenue of $38.5 million or less. This estimate may overstate the actual number of small health insurance companies that would be affected, since almost 74 percent of these small companies belong to larger holding groups, and many, if not all, of these small companies are likely to have non- health lines of business that would result in their revenues exceeding $38.5 million for Direct Health and Medical Insurance Carriers or $32.5 million for HMO Medical Centers.

HHS is not preparing an analysis for the RFA because it has determined, and the Secretary certifies, that this rule will not have a significant economic impact on a substantial number of small entities.

F. Unfunded Mandates

Section 202 of the Unfunded

Mandates Reform Act of 1995 (UMRA) requires that agencies assess anticipated costs and benefits and take certain other actions before issuing a rule that includes any Federal mandate that may result in expenditures in any 1 year by State, local, or Tribal governments, in the aggregate, or by the private sector, of $100 million in 1995 dollars, updated annually for inflation. Currently, that threshold is approximately $146 million. Although we have not been able to quantify all costs, we expect the combined impact on State, local, or Tribal governments and the private sector to be below the threshold.

G. *Federalism*

Executive Order 13132 establishes certain requirements that an agency must meet when it promulgates a rule that imposes substantial direct costs on State and local governments, preempts State law, or otherwise has Federalism implications.

In HHS's view, while this final rule will not impose substantial direct requirement costs on State and local governments, this regulation has Federalism implications due to direct effects on the distribution of power and responsibilities among the State and Federal governments relating to determining standards relating to health insurance that is offered in the individual and small group markets. However, HHS anticipates that the Federalism implications (if any) are substantially mitigated because under the statute and this final rule, States have choices regarding the structure, governance, and operations of their Exchanges. This rule strives to increase flexibility for SBEs. For example, we recommend, but do not require, that SBEs engage in pre-enrollment verification with respect to special enrollment periods; and we will defer to State network adequacy reviews provided the States have the authority and the means to conduct network adequacy reviews. Additionally, the PPACA does not require States to establish these programs; if a State elects not to establish any of these programs or is not approved to do so, HHS must establish and operate the programs in that State.

In compliance with the requirement of Executive Order 13132 that agencies examine closely any policies that may have Federalism implications or limit the policy making discretion of the States, HHS has engaged in efforts to consult with and work cooperatively with affected States, including participating in conference calls with and attending conferences of the National Association of Insurance Commissioners, and consulting with State insurance officials on an individual basis.

While developing this rule, HHS attempted to balance the States' interests in regulating health insurance issuers with the need to ensure market stability. By doing so, it is HHS's view that we have complied with the requirements of Executive Order 13132.

H. Congressional Review Act

This rule is subject to the Congressional Review Act provisions of the Small Business Regulatory Enforcement Fairness Act of 1996 (5 U.S.C. 801, *et seq.*), which specifies that before a rule can take effect, the Federal agency promulgating the rule shall submit to each House of the Congress and to the Comptroller General a report containing a copy of the rule along with other specified information, and has been transmitted to Congress and the Comptroller for review.

I. Reducing Regulation and Controlling Regulatory Costs

Executive Order 13771, entitled Reducing Regulation and Controlling Regulatory Costs, was issued on January 30, 2017. Section 2(a) of Executive Order 13771 requires an agency, unless prohibited by law, to identify at least two existing regulations to be repealed when the agency publicly proposes for notice and comment or otherwise promulgates a new regulation. In furtherance of this requirement, section 2(c) of Executive Order 13771 requires that the new incremental costs associated with new regulations shall, to the extent permitted by law, be offset by the elimination of existing costs associated with at least two prior regulations. It has been determined that this final rule does not impose costs that trigger the above requirements of Executive Order 13771.

PART 155 – EXCHANGE ESTABLISHMENT STANDARDS AND OTHER RELATED STANDARDS UNDER THE AFFORDABLE CARE ACT

§155.400   Enrollment of qualified individuals into QHPs.

*   *   *   *   *

(e) * * *
(1) * * *
(iv) Notwithstanding the requirements in paragraphs (e)(1)(i) through (iii) of this section, for coverage to be effectuated after pended enrollment due to special enrollment period eligibility verification, the binder payment must consist of the premium due for all months of retroactive coverage through the first prospective month of coverage consistent with the coverage effective dates described in §155.420(b)(1),

(2) and (3) or, if elected, §155.420(b)(5) and the deadline for making the binder payment must be no earlier than 30 calendar days from the date the issuer receives the enrollment transaction.

* * * *

■ 5. Section 155.410 is amended by revising paragraphs (e)(2) and (3) to read as follows:

§155. 410   Initial and annual open enrollment periods.

* * * *

(e) * * *

For the benefit years beginning on January 1, 2016 and January 1, 2017, the annual open enrollment period begins on November 1 of the calendar year preceding the benefit year, and extends through January 31 of the benefit year.

For the benefit years beginning on or after January 1, 2018, the annual open enrollment period begins on November 1 and extends through December 15 of the calendar year preceding the benefit year.

* * * * *

■ 6. Section 155.420 is amended by: ■ a. Adding paragraph headings for paragraphs (a)(1) and (2); ■ b. Adding paragraphs (a)(3) through (5);

■ c. Revising paragraphs (b)(1) introductory text, (b)(5), and (d) introductory text; ■ d. Adding paragraph (d)(2)(i)(A) and reserved paragraph (d)(2)(i)(B); and ■ e. Revising paragraph (d)(7).

The additions and revisions read as follows:

§155.420 Special enrollment periods.

(a) * * *
(1)   *General parameters.* * * *
Definition of dependent. * * * (3) *Use of special enrollment periods.* Except in the circumstances specified in paragraph (a)(4) of this section, the Exchange must allow a qualified individual or enrollee, and when specified in paragraph (d) of this section, his or her dependent to enroll in

a QHP if one of the triggering events specified in paragraph (d) of this section occur.

(4) *Use of special enrollment periods by enrollees.* (i) If an enrollee has gained a dependent in accordance with paragraph (d)(2)(i) of this section, the Exchange must allow the enrollee to add the dependent to his or her current QHP, or, if the current QHP's business rules do not allow the dependent to enroll, the Exchange must allow the enrollee and his or her dependents to change to another QHP within the same level of coverage (or one metal level higher or lower, if no such QHP is available), as outlined in §156.140(b) of this subchapter, or, at the option of the enrollee or dependent, enroll the dependent in any separate QHP.

(ii) If an enrollee and his or her dependents become newly eligible for cost-sharing reductions in accordance with paragraph (d)(6)(i) or (ii) of this section and are not enrolled in a silver- level QHP, the Exchange must allow the enrollee and his or her dependents to change to a silver-level QHP if they elect to change their QHP enrollment.

(iii) If an enrollee qualifies for a special enrollment period or is adding a dependent to his or her QHP through a triggering event specified in paragraph (d) of this section other than those described under paragraph (d)(2)(i), (d)(4), (d)(6)(i), (d)(6)(ii), (d)(8), (d)(9), or (d)(10), the Exchange must allow the enrollee and his or her dependents to make changes to his or her enrollment in the same QHP or to change to another QHP within the same level of coverage (or one metal level higher or lower, if no such QHP is available), as outlined in §156.140(b) of this subchapter, or, at the option of the enrollee or dependent, enroll in any separate QHP.

(5) *Prior coverage requirement.* Qualified individuals who are required to demonstrate coverage in the 60 days prior to a qualifying event can either demonstrate that they had minimum essential coverage as described in 26 CFR 1.5000A-1(b) for 1 or more days during the 60 days preceding the date of the qualifying event; lived in a foreign country or in a United States territory for 1 or more days during the 60 days preceding the date of the qualifying event; or that they are an Indian as defined by section 4 of the Indian Health Care Improvement Act.

(b) * * *

(1) *Regular effective dates.* Except as specified in paragraphs (b)(2), (3), and (5) of this section, for a QHP selection received by the Exchange from a qualified individual—

* * *

(5) *Option for later coverage effective dates due to prolonged eligibility verification.* At the option of the consumer, the Exchange must provide for a coverage effective date that is no more than 1 month later than the effective date specified in this paragraph (b) if a consumer's enrollment is delayed until after the verification of the consumer's eligibility for a special enrollment period, and the assignment of a coverage effective date consistent with this paragraph (b) would result in the consumer being required to pay 2 or more months of retroactive premium to effectuate coverage or avoid cancellation.

* * * * *

(d) *Triggering events.* Subject to paragraphs (a)(3) through (5) of this section, as applicable, the Exchange must allow a qualified individual or enrollee, and, when specified below, his or her dependent, to enroll in or change from one QHP to another if one of the triggering events occur:

* * * * *

(2) * * *

(i) * * *

(A) In the case of marriage, at least one spouse must demonstrate having minimum essential coverage as described in 26 CFR 1.5000A-1(b) for 1 or more days during the 60 days preceding the date of marriage. (B) [Reserved]

* * * * *

(7) The qualified individual or enrollee, or his or her dependent, gains access to new QHPs as a result of a permanent move and—

(i) Had minimum essential coverage as described in 26 CFR 1.5000A-1(b) for one or more days during the 60 days preceding the date of the permanent move.

(ii) [Reserved]

* * * *

■ 7. Section 155.725 is amended by adding paragraph (j)(7) to read as follows:

§155.725 Enrollment periods under SHOP.

* * * *

(j) * * *

(7) Notwithstanding anything to the contrary in §155.420(d), §155.420(a)(4) and (d)(2)(i)(A) do not apply to special enrollment periods in the SHOP.

* * * * *

PART 156 — HEALTH INSURANCE ISSUER STANDARDS UNDER THE AFFORDABLE CARE ACT, INCLUDING STANDARDS RELATED TO EXCHANGES

§156.140 Levels of coverage.

* * * * *

(c) *De minimis variation.* For plan years beginning on or after January 1, 2018, the allowable variation in the AV of a health plan that does not result in a material difference in the true dollar value of the health plan is ¥4 percentage points and +2 percentage points, except if a health plan under paragraph (b)(1) of this section (a bronze health plan) either covers and pays for at least one major service, other than preventive services, before the deductible or meets the requirements to be a high deductible health plan within the meaning of 26 U.S.C. 223(c)(2), in which case the allowable variation in AV for such plan is ¥4 percentage points and +5 percentage points.

CMS-9929-P

   Dated: April 10, 2017.

Seema Verma,

Administrator, Centers for Medicare & Medicaid Services.

   Dated: April 11, 2017.

Thomas E. Price,

Secretary, Department of Health and Human Services.

[FR Doc. 2017-07712 Filed 4-13-17; 4:15 pm]

HOW WOULD REPEAL OF OBAMACARE AFFECT YOU

Many people[73] hate that the A.C.A. requires people to buy health insurance or pay a penalty. But without the mandate, fewer younger and healthier people would buy coverage. This would lead to what health experts call a "death spiral" as insurers raise rates because they are left covering people who are older and sicker, leading to even more people dropping coverage. Eventually, companies could stop selling policies directly to individuals in much of the country.

People with individual market coverage: Americans who buy insurance on their own disproportionately benefit from the Affordable Care Act (ACA). They receive tax credits if eligible, enhanced consumer protections, and a transparent Marketplace to buy coverage. Subsequently, these people would disproportionately lose under TrumpCare. The legislation would reduce financial assistance for low- and middle-income enrollees and significantly raise premiums for older enrollees. TrumpCare's state waivers would undermine protections for people with pre-existing conditions. And, it would increase deductibles and cost sharing by eliminating cost sharing subsidies and standards for plans. As such, people who buy coverage on their own and through the Marketplace would pay more out of pocket under TrumpCare.

People with Medicaid: The AHCA would roll back the ACA's expansion of Medicaid, which improved coverage, access to care, and financial security for millions of Americans. Moreover, TrumpCare would cap federal Medicaid funding for every state. This cap would apply to spending for all enrollees, including children needing special education, seniors needing long-term services, people with severe disabilities, and low-income families. By cutting federal spending by one-fourth by 2024, the AHCA would make it virtually impossible for states to manage costs without reducing benefits or coverage altogether for tens of millions of Medicaid enrollees. And by ending retroactive coverage and presumptive eligibility, the AHCA would limit coverage for every person newly enrolling in Medicaid. In short, Medicaid enrollees would lose coverage and benefits under AHCA.

People with employer coverage: The AHCA would eliminate the employer shared-responsibility provision, which currently requires large employers to offer affordable health coverage to their workers, causing some employers to drop coverage altogether. It also would delay implementation of the excise tax on high-cost plans (known as the "Cadillac tax") designed to lower premiums for workers and their families. By allowing states to waive essential health benefits, employers could reduce protections against high annual out-of-pocket costs and lifetime limits on coverage for up to 27 million Americans. And because of the magnitude of coverage losses under the AHCA, every hospital would likely experience spikes in uncompensated care. These costs—which start when an uninsured person walks into the emergency room—could be partially passed along to employer health plans in the form of higher premiums, sometimes called a "hidden tax." As such, TrumpCare would raise costs for people with employer-based health insurance.

People with Medicare: Despite the president's promise not to touch Medicare, TrumpCare does so in several ways. First, the AHCA would repeal an important tax on high-income Americans that supports Medicare. Second, by increasing the number of uninsured Americans, it would increase Medicare's payments for uncompensated care. Third, by capping Medicaid payments for seniors who are also enrolled in Medicare, the legislation could result in cutbacks for services such as home care, driving up Medicare-financed services like hospitalizations. And, fourth, by repealing the drug industry fee whose revenue is dedicated to Medicare Part B, the bill would raise the program's premiums by $8.7 billion over ten years. The AHCA would take two years off of the life of the Medicare Hospital Insurance Trust Fund, according to its actuaries. As such, TrumpCare would harm all seniors by raising Medicare premiums and making the Medicare Trust Fund bankrupt in less than a decade.

The legislation's impact does not end there. It would also affect people who get health care through the Veterans Health Administration: 7 million people would no longer would be able to access premium tax credits through the Marketplace. People insured through private plans in TriCare may also pay higher premiums to offset rising levels of uninsurance. And the AHCA's Medicaid cuts could limit support for the Indian Health Services.

Notably, the one group of Americans that TrumpCare would explicitly exempt is members of Congress. They would maintain pre-existing condition protections.

There is no "us versus them" in this debate over health care. If the AHCA is signed into law, health coverage could be worse for us all.

OBAMACARE-TRUMPCARE

HEALTHCARE FOR PRISONERS

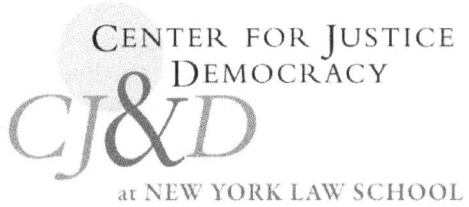

CENTER FOR JUSTICE &
DEMOCRACY 185 WEST
BROADWAY
NEW YORK, NY 10013

FAQ – CIVIL JUSTICE AND PRISON HEALTH CARE: ALL LOCKED UP AND BEHIND BARS

Do sick and injured inmates have a right to health care while incarcerated?

Yes. The U.S. Supreme Court has long recognized that prisoners have a constitutional right to adequate health care through the Eighth Amendment's ban on "cruel and unusual" punishment. To constitute an Eighth Amendment violation, prison personnel must act with "deliberate indifference to serious medical needs of prisoners." However, like any patient, inmates have the right to be treated in a non-negligent manner. In other words, even if inadequate health care does not rise to the level of a constitutional violation, state negligence standards still may be violated. Enforcing these rights in court, however, can be very difficult for inmates.

How does a prisoner receive health care?

There are three possible scenarios:

1) The prison is government-run, with the government providing health care. The prison is government-run, with the government outsourcing health care to a private contractor. As reported by *Prison Legal News*, "Around 20 states outsource all or some of the

medical services in their prison systems," while the federal government outsources some aspects of health-care operations in its facilities.

2) The prison is corporate-run, with a private company operating the inmate health care system. As of 2013, private prisons held 19 percent of federal prisoners and 7 percent of state prisoners. This population is increasing. From 2000-2013, the number of state and federal prisoners in private prisons rose by more than 46 percent (from 90,815 in 2000 to 133,000 in 2013). When looking solely at federal prisoners in private prisons, the numbers more than doubled, going from 15,524 in 2000 to 41,159 in 2013.

Why would governments turn to private prison companies to provide health care services?

Cost Savings. State and federal budgets are being strained by the exploding prison populations. This rapid growth is often attributed to "a series of 'get tough' policies enacted in the 1980s and into the 1990s, such as truth in sentencing laws, mandatory minimums, mandatory drug sentences, life sentence without possibility of parole, and the three-strikes law." Along with prison population growth comes the accompanying cost of providing health care for inmates (many of whom enter prison with chronic illnesses, infectious diseases and other health problems). In addition, the number of inmates over the age of 55 is rising, increasing 234 percent between 1999 to 2013. The cost to treat these patients is, on average, at least 2-3 times that of other inmates.[1]

Outsourcing health care to private prison health care companies, which are predicated on a cost-cutting model to boost profits, may sound appealing to cash-strapped governments despite what it might mean for the quality of care provided. Some contracts require specific cuts in health care costs, such as the five-year contract between Florida's Department of Corrections (FDOC) and Corizon, the nation's largest for-profit prison health care provider, where the company agreed to provide the current quality of medical care to Florida state prisoners for 7 percent less than it cost the FDOC.

Reduced accountability. Outsourcing prison health care allows governments to transfer some or all of their legal liability to private contractors when inmates suffer medical injuries. On a related note, prison health care privatization can enable governments to essentially hand off oversight responsibilities relating to the provision and quality of medical services. However, governments are not always "off the hook" when outsourced or private health care is inadequate. State officials, in particular, can sometimes be held jointly responsible when a private company has been "deliberately indifferent to serious medical needs of prisoners."

Can private health care be unsafe for prisoners?

Yes. Whether it is due to cost cutting or simple disregard for inmates' well-being, health care for prisoners is often abysmal and can be deadly. This problem permeates every part of the country.

For example, from January 2013 through May 2014 in Illinois, there were "significant lapses in care" in an "unacceptably high" 60 percent of the cases in which state prisoners died of natural causes. This was the finding of an independent report submitted by medical experts in connection with a class action lawsuit that alleged unsafe medical care at the state's prisons, care provided to roughly 50,000 inmates by Wexford Health under a 10-year, $1.36 billion contract. The report uncovered serious problems with treatment of ordinary illnesses, such as a doctor stopping a diabetic patient's insulin treatment "after his blood sugar levels were found to be normal while he was on the insulin," an inmate's foot being amputated after a "grossly mismanaged" ulcer and a prisoner who was sent to the hospital two weeks after a "rapidly progressive paralysis of the lower half of his body," leaving him in a wheelchair.

A recent investigation in Arizona uncovered "disturbing cases of inadequate treatment" by private prison health care companies Corizon and Wexford Health Sources in state prisons. According to a former Corizon patient care technician, staffing levels left dementia patients unfed, incontinent inmates sitting for hours in their own feces and other prisoners dead. In one case, a pregnant inmate in jail on drug charges was forced to have a cesarean delivery and quickly moved back to her cell where her wound re-opened. She alerted prison staff but was refused medical attention. When she was finally able to see medical staff two weeks later, they then treated her with a "wound vacuum" and table sugar – an antiquated treatment used before the invention of antibiotics.

In Florida, according to a *Palm Beach Post* investigation, "Just months after all medical care in state prisons was privatized, the count of inmate deaths spiked to a 10-year high in January [2014] and continued at a record pace through July." Among the countless victims of life threatening health care: a 24-year-old Florida man, in jail for a misdemeanor, who alerted health care workers after he felt "his intestines escaping from his rectum." As reported by the *Miami Herald,* "Fellow inmates begged Corizon's staff to take him to a hospital" but instead the Corizon nurse "'obtained some K-Y Jelly, and pushed the intestines back in,'" civil court records show. "Hours later, at a local hospital, doctors found an abscess compressing his spine."

In 2015, Corizon was fired by New York City after its Department of Investigation (DOI) discovered that the "company had hired doctors and mental health workers with disciplinary problems and criminal convictions, including for murder and kidnapping. It also found that missteps by Corizon employees might have contributed to at least two recent inmate deaths." In one case, "an inmate was left dying, untreated for six days while uniformed officers, doctors, mental health clinicians and nurses made 57 visits to his cell without assisting him."

What can a prisoner do legally if he or she has been provided unsafe health care?

Before harmed federal inmates can even file a lawsuit, they must first jump through administrative hurdles established by the Prisoners Reform Litigation Act (PLRA). Many states have passed versions of the PLRA, which similarly obstruct state court access. Once those obstacles are overcome, an inmate's legal options depend on three main factors: 1) whether s/he is in local, state or federal prison; 2) whether the health care is provided by the government or a private company; and 3) the degree of harm inflicted.

What if an inmate is provided inadequate health care in a *federal* facility?

Health care provided by the government. If a federal inmate's harm is caused by "deliberate indifference to a serious medical need," this mistreatment may violate the U.S. Constitution's Eighth Amendment prohibition against cruel and unusual punishment. That may give rise to a "constitutional tort" also known as a *"Bivens"* action, allowing a lawsuit against prison officials (but not against the federal government itself). "Deliberate indifference" is a much higher standard than "negligence" or "malpractice," requiring "more than ordinary lack of due care."

If the harms committed against the inmate do not rise to the level of a constitutional violation the inmate may still be able to bring a malpractice claim under the Federal Tort Claims Act (FTCA). The FTCA allows federal prisoners (without regard to citizenship status) assigned to publicly-run prison facilities to file a tort claim against the United States when a federal employee has injured them. Before a claim can be filed under the FTCA, the inmate must exhaust administrative remedies by first filing a complaint with the Bureau of Prisons. There are also strict limits on the kinds of damages they may recover.

Health care provided by a private company. If a federal inmate happens to be housed in a privately-run federal prison, or his or her health care is provided by a private contractor, his or her rights completely change. The Supreme Court has said that *Bivens* actions are not available to federal inmates in private prisons as long as state tort law provides an alternative remedy, irrespective of how sufficient that remedy may be. In addition, federal prisoners held at privately-run facilities cannot sue under the FTCA because contractors are not federal employees for purposes of the Act. However, as the Supreme Court has suggested, remedies against private companies may still be available under state tort law.

What if an inmate is provided inadequate health care in a *state or local* facility?

If a state or local inmate's harm is caused by "deliberate indifference to a serious medical need," this mistreatment may violate the U.S. Constitution's Eighth Amendment prohibition against cruel and unusual punishment. In that case, inmates can pursue a civil rights action in federal court under 42 U.S.C Sec. 1983. While a state government cannot be sued under Section 1983, state and local officials can be sued. (If found liable, the state will usually indemnify their employee.) In addition, *private* health care contractors and their employees can be sued under Section 1983. In fact, a state official and private contractor may be jointly liable for causing harm.

If a claim does not rise to the level of a constitutional violation, a private prison official may be liable under state medical malpractice law. Cases against the state are more difficult because of sovereign immunity issues. Most states have some kind of state tort claims act modeled on the FTCA, waiving sovereign immunity to some extent and allowing some claims to proceed.

However, these laws typically have administration requirements and contain liability limits.

What additional obstacles do prisoners face in accessing the civil justice system and what are the ramifications?

Inmates face a number of other difficulties bringing lawsuits over inadequate or dangerous health care. For example, because they are incarcerated, inmates' damages may be extremely low and juries may be unsympathetic. Noted one New Mexico attorney, culpable defendants may refuse to settle a prisoner's case, "argu[ing] that inmates' damages are minimal since they can't factor in lost wages. That leaves the option of a jury trial, but jurors tend to take a dim view of inmate complaints."

Similarly, an Illinois attorney explained that "low settlements discourage lawyers from taking cases." Another stated, "The economic incentives of the entities that are entrusted is to give as little care as possible.... They're in an industry where they don't think they will be scrutinized. Even if the worst-case scenario happens, juries won't care that much. So they are emboldened."

Because civil lawsuits may be the only means to hold private prison operators, private health care contractors and their employees and government officials accountable for providing dangerous medical care, the scarcity of lawsuits has likely led to even worse conditions. Lawsuits are often the only means for the public and government regulators to learn about unsafe medical practices in the nation's prisons. This is especially true for private contractor-operated prisons, which, in contrast to government-run federal and state facilities, are under no obligation to be transparent about the level and quality of prisoner health care. Sometimes it takes repeated litigation and the accompanying publicity to push a legislature to act or force a government agency to implement stronger regulations, exercise greater oversight or terminate a prison health care contract.

INDEX

ABORTIONS, 19, 20
ABOUT OBAMACARE, 3
ABSTINENCE, 21
ACA, 6, 7, 8, 9, 10, 11, 12, 50, 51, 157
Active living, 4
Afford, 13
benefits, 5, 8, 9, 10, 12, 19, 23, 29, 30, 31, 32, 33, 37, 38, 39, 40, 41, 42, 45, 47, 49, 157
BENEFITS, 29, 30, 37, 45, 49
BIRTH, 20
Catastrophic, 12, 32
childbirth, 8, 10, 20, 21
children, 6, 10, 18, 24, 25, 38, 39, 40, 157
CHOICE, 19, 25, 30, 31, 37, 39
chronic illness, 5
chronically, 6
community, 10, 13, 25, 26, 27, 28, 29, 33, 49
CONSUMER, 30, 32
copayments, 6, 13
costs, 3, 5, 6, 7, 8, 9, 10, 13, 26, 32, 38, 51, 52, 157
deductibles, 7, 13, 39, 157
DENTAL, 29, 45
deny coverage, 6
denying health coverage, 6
DEPENDENT, 38
dialysis services., 7
DISEASE, 36
doctor, 5, 9, 11
drop, 6, 8, 157
DUAL, 41

EDUCATION, 15, 16, 21
elder abuse., **4**
emergency room, **5**, **7**, **8**, **10**, **13**, **158**
employees, 5, 8, 9, 10, 12, 13, 30, 50
end-of-life, 11
exchanges, 7, 9, 10, 12, 13
family, 6, 7, 13, 15, 21, 26, 27, 29, 32, 33, 37, 38
FAMILY PLANNING, 21
financial, 4, 12, 13, 16, 28, 47, 49, 157
financial interest, **4**
FRAUD, 41
GUARANTEED, 35, 36
gynecological, 19
health care providers and high-income families, 3
health insurance, 3, 5, 6, 7, 8, 10, 12, 13, 18, 23, 24, 31, 34, 35, 36, 37, 40, 41, 43, 46, 50, 51, 52, 156, 158
HEALTH STATUS, 36
Healthy eating, 4
high-risk providers, **4**
home health agencies, 7
Home health care, 9
hospice, 9
hospitals, 4, 7, 10, 51
immigrants, 10, 38
IMMUNIZATIONS, 23
income, 3, 4, 7, 8, 10, 11, 12, 13, 21, 25, 33, 44, 46, 48, 50, 51, 52, 157, 158
information, 7, 9, 14, 15, 23, 28, 29, 33, 36, 42, 43, 47
Injury and violence-free living, **4**
insured, **5**, **158**

INDEX

limit, 6, 32, 38, 39, 157, 158
LIMITS, 31
LONG TERM, 25
mammograms, 9
maternity, 8
Medicaid, 3, 5, 6, 7, 8, 10, 12, 13, 17, 18, 27, 40, 41, 49, 51, 52, 157, 158
medical coverage, 5
medical services, 6
Medicare, 3, 4, 5, 7, 8, 9, 11, 12, 17, 18, 41, 50, 158
medications, 7
Mental and emotional health, 4
middle-income families, 3, 8
NONDISCRIMINATION, 47
nursing home staff, 4
nursing homes, 4, 7
Obamacare, 1, 3, 5, 6, 7, 8, 9, 10, 11, 12, 14, 22, 49, 50, 51, 52
OBSTETRICAL, 18
PEDIATRIC, 24, 45
penalty, 9, 12, 41, 47, 50, 156
physically challenged, 4
physicals, 9
physicians, 4, 7, 29
plans, 5, 6, 7, 8, 9, 12, 13, 14, 17, 19, 32, 33, 35, 37, 38, 39, 40, 42, 43, 44, 50, 51, 157, 158
poverty, 13, 25, 44
POWER OF ATTORNEY, 16
pre-existing condition, 5, 35, 38, 39, 158
pregnancy, 6, 8, 15
premiums, 4, 5, 6, 7, 8, 33, 38, 44, 50, 157, 158
prescriptions, 7

Preventing drug abuse and excessive alcohol use, **4**
PREVENTION, 17, 34, 36
preventive, 9, 10, 18, 25, 43
primary, 4, 10, 18, 24, 32, 37
private, 5, 8, 13, 40, 158
QUALITY, 34
RELIGIOUS, 45
repeal, 51, 158
Reproductive and sexual health., **4**
Republicans, 49, 51, 52
RESCISSIONS, 31
retiree, 12
scholarships and loans, **4**
self-employed, 5
skilled nursing services, 9
smoke, 10
smoking, 10, 28
state exchanges, **4**
STATES, 30, 40, 48
subsidies, 3, 5, 7, 12, 13, 20, 33, 40, 47, 157
test, 4, 9, 16
THERAPIES, 14
Tobacco-free living, **4**
treatment, 1, 5, 8, 9, 13, 14, 15, 16, 19, 21, 24, 49
TRUMP CARE, 49
Trumpcare, 50, 51
Wellness, **6, 34**
WELLNESS, 17, 34
women, 8, 14, 18, 22, 23, 51
WOMEN, 18, 22
workers, 9, 11, 12, 157

REFERENCES

[1] See "AN INEXPLICABLE DEFORMITY" ISBN: and "REMEDY AND REDEMPTION" ISBN:

[2] As provided for by DHS

[3] I have modified the text and added to demonstrate my point.

[4] **SEC. 1554**

[5] **SEC. 513**

[6] **SEC. 2955.**

[7] **SEC. 3113**

[8] **SEC. 2301.**

[9] SEC. 1920C

[10] **SEC. 2954.**

[11] **SEC. 925**

[12] **SEC. 713**

[13] SEC. 1001\2714

[14] **SEC. 2402.**

[15] **SEC. 2501.**

[16] **SEC. 2503**

REFERENCES

[17] **SEC. 2703.**

[18] **SEC. 1312 o42 U.S.C. 18032**

[19] SEC. 2711 o42 U.S.C. 300gg–11..

[20] SEC. 2711 o42 U.S.C. 300gg–11..

[21] SEC. 2712 o42 U.S.C. 300gg–12..

[22] FPL Federal Poverty Level

[23] SEC. 2717 o42 U.S.C. 300gg–17..

[24] SEC. 2719 o42 U.S.C. 300gg–19..

[25] SEC. 1101 o42 U.S.C. 18001

[26] SEC. 2702 o42 U.S.C. 300gg–1..

[27] 'SEC. 2703 o42 U.S.C. 300gg–2..

[28] SEC. 2705 o42 U.S.C. 300gg–4..

[29] **"SEC. 2708 o42 U.S.C. 300gg–7..**

[30] **SEC. 1331 o42 U.S.C. 18051..**

[31] **SEC. 36B.**

[32] **113 PPACA**

[33] **SEC. 1555**

[34] **SEC. 1557**

REFERENCES

[35] SEC. 1558.

[36] This is an excerpt from a posting on the web whose author I am unable to find. I have modified the text and added to demonstrate my point. LifeDaily.com

[37] The HIPAA requirement for guaranteed renewability, codified in section 2712 of the PHS Act, was renumbered by the PPACA to section 2703 of the PHS Act. HIPAA's guaranteed renewability requirement continues to apply in certain contexts, such as to issuers in the U.S. territories and issuers of expatriate health plans.

[38] Initial Guidance to States on Exchanges (November 10, 2018). Available at *https:// www.cms.gov/CCIIO/Resources/Files/guidance_to_states_on_exchanges.html.*

[39] Similar provisions in §146.150 apply to health insurance issuers offering grandfathered and non- grandfathered coverage in the small group market.

[40] For purposes of this rulemaking, the term "past- due premiums" refers to premiums that have not been paid by the applicable due date as established by the issuer in accordance with applicable Federal and State law. It does not include premiums for months in which individuals were not enrolled in coverage.

[41] Federally-facilitated Marketplace (FFM) and Federally-facilitated Small Business Health Options Program Enrollment Manual, Section 6.3 Terminations for Non-Payment of Premiums, available at *https://www.cms.gov/CCIIO/Resources/ Regulations-and-Guidance/Downloads/ENR_ FFMSHOP_Manual_080916.pdf.*

[42] *See* summary of comments at 78 FR 13416 (Feb. 27, 2013).

[43] Issuers may also have obligations under other applicable Federal laws prohibiting discrimination, and issuers are responsible for ensuring compliance with all applicable laws and regulations.

[44] As discussed below, the FF–SHOP is unable to offer issuers this flexibility at this time.

[45] For example, a subscriber of an individual policy or an employer that purchases a group policy is typically responsible for payment of the

REFERENCES

premiums. Thus, an issuer cannot refuse to effectuate new coverage purchased by a dependent because the subscriber owes past-due premiums or new coverage purchased by a current or former employee (or his or her dependent) because the employee's employer owes past-due premiums.

[46] *See* 45 CFR 147.106(d)(4). States adopting the policy may use a narrower definition of "controlled group.

[47] *FFM and FFM–SHOP Enrollment Manual* (Section 6.1).

[48] See 81 FR 12274.

[49] November 2016, *Results of Enrollment Testing for the 2016 Special Enrollment Period,* GAO–17– 78, US Government Accountability Office.

[50] February 25, 2016, Fact Sheet: Special Enrollment Confirmation Process. Available online at https://www.cms.gov/Newsroom/MediaReleaseDatabase/Fact-sheets/2016-Fact- sheets-items/2016-02-24.html.

[51] Ibid.

[52] December 14, 2016, Fact Sheet: Pre-Enrollment Verification for Special Enrollment Periods, available at https://www.cms.gov/CCIIO/Resources/Fact-Sheets-and-FAQs/Downloads/Pre-Enrollment- SEP-fact-sheet-FINAL.PDF.

[53] Stan Dorn, Enrollment Periods in 2015 and Beyond: Potential Effects on Enrollment and Program Administration (Washington, DC: Urban Institute, February 2015), available online at http://www.urban.org/sites/default/files/publication/ 41616/2000104-Enrollment-Periods-in-2015-and- Beyond.pdf.

[54] Centers for Medicare and Medicaid Services (CMS), Pre-Enrollment Verification

[55] HHS, *Clarifying, Eliminating and Enforcing Special Enrollment Periods* (January 19, 2016), available at http://wayback.archive-it.org/2744/20170118130449/https://blog.cms.gov/2016/01/19/ clarifying-eliminating-and-enforcing-special- enrollment-periods/.

[56] Key Dates for Calendar Year 2017: Qualified

REFERENCES

Health Plan Certification in the Federally-facilitated Exchanges; Rate Review; Risk Adjustment and Reinsurance, (April 2017), available at https:// www.cms.gov/CCIIO/Resources/Regulations-and-Guidance/index.html#.

[57] Available at https://www.cms.gov/CCIIO/ Resources/Files/Downloads/Av-csr-bulletin.pdf.

[58] Although we proposed to expand the de minimis range for bronze plans to ¥4 percentage points, we also recognized that achieving an AV below 58 percent is difficult with the claims distribution underlying the current AV Calculator.

[59] As of the 2018 plan year, no State has an AV Calculator that utilizes state-specific data under §156.135(e); therefore, an AV Calculator that utilizes State-specific data is intended for plan years beyond 2018.

[60] For the purposes of this section of the rule, references to decreases in APTCs also reflect the possibility of decreases in premium tax credits not paid in advance.

[61] A plan with a deductible of $7,350 that is equal to the annual limitation on cost sharing of $7,350 for 2018 with no services covered until the deductible and annual limitation on cost sharing are met, other than preventive services required to be covered without cost sharing under section 2713 of the PHS Act and §147.130, has an AV of 58.54 percent based on the 2018 AV Calculator. 81 FR 61455. September 6, 2016.

[62] A Revised Final 2018 AV Calculator, User Guide and Methodology are posted on CCIIO's Web site under "Plan Management" at https:// www.cms.gov/cciio/resources/regulations-and- guidance/#Plan Management.

[63] Letter to Issuers on Federally-facilitated and State Partnership Exchanges (April 5, 2013). Available at https://www.cms.gov/CCIIO/Resources/ Regulations-and-Guidance/Downloads/2014_letter_ to_issuers_04052013.pdf.

[64] Recognition of Entities for the Accreditation of Qualified Health Plans 77 FR 70163 (November 23, 2013and Approval of an Application by the

REFERENCES

[65] Accreditation Association for Ambulatory Health Care (AAAHC) To Be a Recognized Accrediting Entity for the Accreditation of Qualified Health Plans 78 FR 77470 (December 23 2013,).

[66] The National Association of Insurance Commissioners' Health Benefit Plan Network Access and Adequacy Model Act is available at http://www.naic.org/store/free/MDL-74.pdf.

[67] Key Dates for Calendar Year 2017: QHP Certification in the Federally-facilitated Marketplaces; Rate Review; Risk Adjustment and Reinsurances, Revised February 2017, *available at* https://www.cms.gov/CCIIO/Resources/Regulations- and-Guidance/Downloads/Revised-Key-Dates-for- Calendar-Year-2017-2-17-17.pdf.

[68] Letter to Issuers in the Federally- facilitated Marketplaces. Available at https:// www.cms.gov/CCIIO/Resources/Regulations-and-Guidance/Downloads/2015-final-issuer-letter-3-14- 2014.pdf.

[69] List available at https://www.cms.gov/CCIIO/ Programs-and-Initiatives/Health-Insurance- Marketplaces/Downloads/FINAL-CMS-ECP-LIST- PY-2018_12-16-16.xlsx.

[70] For a list of types of providers eligible to participate in the 340B Drug Program, *see* https:// www.hrsa.gov/opa/eligibilityandregistration/ index.html.

[71] As some commenters noted, preliminary data regarding HHS's special enrollment confirmation process did indicate a decrease in special enrollment period plan selection. See, Frequently Asked Questions Regarding Verification of Special Enrollment Periods (Sept. 6, 2016) *available at* https://www.cms.gov/CCIIO/Resources/Regulations- and-Guidance/Downloads/FAQ-Regarding- Verification-of-SEPs.pdf.

[72] "Table of Small Business Size Standards Matched to North American Industry Classification System Codes", effective February 26, 2016, U.S. Small Business Administration, available at https:// www.sba.gov/contracting/getting-started-contractor/ make-sure-you-meet-sba-size-standards/table- small-business-size-standards.

REFERENCES

[73] State Coverage Estimates: Estimates for state Medicare, Medicaid, and employer-sponsored insurance were taken from 2015 data from the Kaiser Family Foundation State Health Facts. Estimates for the number of Marketplace enrollees were obtained from the 2015 Marketplace Enrollment Report from HHS. Note that those enrolled in both Medicaid and Medicare are categorized in the Medicaid enrollment and not in Medicare enrollment. State Coverage Loss Estimates: Estimates for 2026 coverage loss (increase in the uninsured) were obtained from the Center for American Progress and based on the Congressional Budget Office's estimate of 23 million in that year.County Coverage Estimates: Data by county from the 2015 American Community Survey from the U.S. Census were obtained to estimate Medicare, Medicaid, and employer-sponsored insurance coverage estimates. For data consistency, the county coverage data were used to calculate relative state-based weights for each county and were scaled to state totals used in the state map. Estimates for Marketplace enrollment by county for 2017 were obtained from the Kaiser Family Foundation and similarly used to calculate county-based weights for application to total state 2015 Marketplace enrollment.

County Coverage Loss Estimates: Our county estimates follow the analytic and data approach taken by the Center for American Progress, with data from the American Community Survey from the U.S. Census at the county rather than congressional district level. Note that the American Community Survey uses a different number of years to estimate county rather than congressional district coverage.

Coverage Loss Risk Estimates: States and counties were divided up into three categories—low, medium, and high—based on the percentage of the total population under age 65 represented by the estimated AHCA's coverage losses by geographic area.

Note, all numbers rounded and may not sum to totals.

The House separately passed bills to remove the exemption for Members of Congress from the state waivers of community rating and essential health benefits and restore Veterans' access to tax credits.

www.ingramcontent.com/pod-product-compliance
Lightning Source LLC
Chambersburg PA
CBHW051549020426
42333CB00016B/2178